T0243088

# Marketing in Healthcare-Related Industries

# Marketing in Healthcare-Related Industries

## Robert E. Hinson
*University of Ghana Business School*

## Ogechi Adeola
*Lagos Business School, Pan-Atlantic University, Nigeria*

## Yam B. Limbu
*Montclair State University, United States of America*

## Emmanuel Mogaji
*University of Greenwich, United Kingdom*

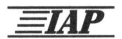

INFORMATION AGE PUBLISHING, INC.
Charlotte, NC • www.infoagepub.com

**Library of Congress Cataloging-in-Publication Data**

A CIP record for this book is available from the Library of Congress
http://www.loc.gov

ISBN: 978-1-64802-106-0 (Paperback)
   978-1-64802-107-7 (Hardcover)
   978-1-64802-108-4 (E-Book)

Printed in the United States of America

# Contents

Foreword.................................................................................... xi

Preface.................................................................................... xiii

1  An Introduction to Marketing in Healthcare................................. 1
    Chapter Outline.................................................................... 1
    Chapter Outcome ................................................................. 1
    Introduction ........................................................................ 2
    The History of Marketing: A Conceptual Perspective ................. 5
    Why Healthcare Marketing is Different..................................... 9
    Reasons for the Adoption of Healthcare Marketing................... 15
    Conclusion.......................................................................... 19
    Review Questions ................................................................ 20
    Mini Case Study With Discussion .......................................... 21
    References ........................................................................... 22

2  Services Marketing as the Bedrock of Healthcare Marketing...... 25
    Chapter Outline.................................................................. 25
    Chapter Outcome ............................................................... 26
    Introduction ...................................................................... 26
    Evolution of the Services Marketing Concept: From 4Ps to 7Ps.... 27
    Services in the Modern Economy............................................ 34
    The Importance of Differences Among Services ........................ 37

The Importance of Marketing Healthcare Services.....................38
Integrating Marketing With Other Functions
    in Healthcare Organization.......................................39
Conclusion.............................................................40
Review Questions......................................................41
Mini Case Study With Discussion......................................41
References............................................................42

**3   The Evolving Societal and Healthcare Context.......................... 45**
Chapter Outline.......................................................45
Chapter Outcome.......................................................46
Introduction..........................................................46
The Evolution of Healthcare...........................................47
The Cultural Revolution and Healthcare................................47
The Changing Societal Context.........................................49
The Country Context...................................................52
The Emergence of Healthcare as an Institution.........................53
Marketing Concepts for Healthcare Organizations.......................59
Components of the Healthcare Marketing Mix............................65
Conclusion............................................................70
Review Questions......................................................71
Mini Case Study With Discussion......................................71
References............................................................72

**4   Public Sector Marketing in Healthcare ..................................77**
Chapter Outline.......................................................77
Chapter Outcome.......................................................78
Introduction..........................................................78
Key Characteristics of Public Services................................78
Scope and Nature of Public Sector Marketing...........................80
Importance of Marketing in the Public Sector..........................82
Challenges of Public Sector Marketing.................................83
The Marketing Mix of Public Sector Marketing..........................86
Types of Marketing in the Public Sector...............................90
Aspects of Social Marketing...........................................95
The Public Sector Marketing Planning Process..........................96
Conclusion............................................................98

Review Questions ..................................................................... 99
Mini Case Study With Discussion .................................................. 99
References ........................................................................... 101

**5  Strategic Planning in Healthcare Marketing ..........................105**
Chapter Outline............................................................. 105
Chapter Outcome ......................................................... 106
Introduction ................................................................. 106
Strategic Planning ........................................................ 106
Strategic Analysis ......................................................... 115
Strategy Formulation..................................................... 120
Strategy Implementation................................................ 121
Strategy Evaluation ....................................................... 123
Conclusion.................................................................... 126
Review Questions .......................................................... 126
Mini Case Study With Discussion ..................................... 127
References .................................................................... 129

**6  Managing Innovation in Healthcare Institutions ........................133**
Chapter Outline............................................................. 133
Chapter Outcome ......................................................... 134
Introduction ................................................................. 134
Uncertainty in Healthcare Institutions ............................... 134
Managing Uncertainty in Healthcare Institutions.................. 136
Organizational Structure and Innovations ........................... 136
Flexibility...................................................................... 139
Communication ............................................................. 139
Interorganizational Relationships...................................... 140
Conclusion.................................................................... 140
Review Questions .......................................................... 141
Mini Case Study With Discussion ..................................... 141
References .................................................................... 142

**7  Healthcare Stakeholders ........................................................145**
Chapter Outline............................................................. 145
Chapter Outcome ......................................................... 146
Introduction ................................................................. 146

Who Is a Stakeholder? ................................................................ 147

Stakeholders in Healthcare Sector ........................................... 147

Stakeholder Theory .................................................................... 152

Stakeholder Value ...................................................................... 153

Difference Between a Stakeholder and a Shareholder .............. 155

Stakeholder Identification ......................................................... 155

Generic Stakeholder Identification ........................................... 156

Engagement Guidelines ............................................................. 156

Snowballing ................................................................................ 158

Mapping ..................................................................................... 158

Identifying Stakeholders' Needs ............................................... 160

Managing Value Through Stakeholder Management ............... 161

Sustaining Stakeholder Value ................................................... 163

Managing Sustainable Stakeholder Value ............................... 163

Evaluating the Impact of Stakeholder Value Created .............. 166

Conclusion .................................................................................. 167

Review Questions ....................................................................... 167

Mini Case Study With Discussion ............................................. 168

References .................................................................................. 169

**8  Consumer Behavior in Healthcare Service Encounters .............. 173**

Chapter Outline .......................................................................... 173

Chapter Outcome ....................................................................... 174

Introduction ............................................................................... 174

Consumers' Interactions With Healthcare Service Operators ... 174

The Multiple Steps in the Healthcare Service
 Purchase Process ................................................................... 177

Health Service Customers' Needs and Expectations
 in Relation to Service Offerings ........................................... 180

Disconfirmation Theory ............................................................. 183

Customer Expectation in Products and Services ...................... 184

Monitoring Customer Needs and Expectations Constantly ...... 187

Customer Expectation in Healthcare Services .......................... 189

Expectation of the Aged in Healthcare Services ...................... 189

Service Evaluation by Healthcare Service Customers .............. 190

Cues and Signals of Service Quality ......................................... 191

The Healthcare Service Business as a System............................. 193

Conclusion...................................................................................... 197

Review Questions.......................................................................... 197

Mini Case Study With Discussion .............................................. 198

References ...................................................................................... 198

**9    Positioning Healthcare Services in Competitive Markets ..........205**

Chapter Outline............................................................................. 205

Chapter Outcome ......................................................................... 206

Introduction .................................................................................. 206

Focus Strategy and Competitive Advantage ............................. 206

Internal, Market, and Competitor Analysis .............................. 214

Positioning Maps.......................................................................... 217

How to Effect Changes in Competitive Positioning.................. 219

Conclusion...................................................................................... 221

Review Questions.......................................................................... 221

Mini Case Study With Discussion .............................................. 222

References ...................................................................................... 224

**10   Balancing Healthcare Service Demand and Capacity .................227**

Chapter Outline............................................................................. 227

Chapter Outcome ......................................................................... 228

Introduction .................................................................................. 228

Fluctuations in Demand and Healthcare Service Productivity ... 228

Demand and Capacity of a Healthcare Service Organization..... 233

Managing Demand Levels and Waiting Times........................... 234

Inventory Holding ........................................................................ 237

Inventory Models ......................................................................... 237

Managing Perceptions of Waiting Time .................................... 238

Conclusion...................................................................................... 239

Review Questions.......................................................................... 240

Mini Case Study With Discussion .............................................. 240

References ...................................................................................... 241

**11   Managing Relationships and Building Loyalty
      in Healthcare Industries............................................................245**

Chapter Outline............................................................................. 245

Chapter Outcome .......................................................................... 246

Introduction ................................................................................ 246

Understanding the Customer-Healthcare Firm Relationship ..... 247

Targeting the Customers............................................................... 248

Analyzing and Managing Customer Databases.......................... 250

Building Customer Loyalty .......................................................... 251

Customer Relationship Management in Healthcare Delivery .....254

Conclusion..................................................................................... 258

Review Questions.......................................................................... 258

Mini Case Study With Discussion ............................................... 259

References ..................................................................................... 260

**12  Marketing Tool Kit for Healthcare Managers .............................265**

Chapter Outline............................................................................ 265

Chapter Outcome ........................................................................ 266

Introduction ................................................................................ 266

The Tool Kit ................................................................................. 267

Conclusion..................................................................................... 273

**About the Authors........................................................................275**

# *Foreword*

In addition to seeking treatment and patient care, the present-day population is more aware of preventive measures; this phenomenon had triggered enormous growth in demand for a range of goods and services (e.g., use of wearable technologies, nutrition, Google search, social media). Traditionally, healthcare delivery systems were considered more like a nonprofit service-oriented activity with limited use of marketing strategies; but with the entry of for-profit and privately managed firms, healthcare providers have changed the way marketing is used in healthcare-related industries. In the context of the change, the book, *Marketing in Healthcare-Related Industries* makes an important contribution to academics as well as professionals interested in advancing their knowledge and skills in healthcare marketing.

Since most healthcare services are rendered for a population located within a specific geographic area, people living in specific locations do not only employ the services of health providers located nearby, but they are also likely to share information and experiences with peers from their neighborhoods. In view of the locational factors, healthcare marketers are more likely to capitalize on exploiting marketing methods and strategies that are appropriate for local conditions. Being local, healthcare providers focus more on customer relationship, building a positive image, and sustaining a good relationship with area-based stakeholders. The authors of the book have emphasized the need for innovation to develop and implement appropriate marketing methods and strategies that are relevant to the

*Marketing in Healthcare-Related Industries,* pages xi–xii
Copyright © 2020 by Information Age Publishing
All rights of reproduction in any form reserved.

targeted population. The authors have also highlighted some of the best practices of professionally managed for-profit hospitals located in different countries and no doubt such examples will add value to the publication. In view of the importance of the local markets, the authors have elaborated on the concepts of the marketing mix in the context of segmentation and targeting specific segments using differentiated marketing methods and strategies that would maximize usage rate, revenue, and profitability.

The authors have done an excellent job of integrating their own perspectives and insights drawn from their research and professional experiences in developed as well as developing markets. This book, containing 12 chapters, is well balanced in terms of length and writing style. The authors have also provided an abstract and bibliography, along with review questions and case studies for each chapter. Given the nature of the healthcare market and its complexity, I believe the book, *Marketing in Healthcare-Related Industries* will be a valuable resource for academics engaged in teaching undergraduate and graduate courses in health-related areas and the practitioners will surely find the Marketing Tool Kit for Healthcare quite useful. I commend the authors who have extensive teaching and research experience for having collaborated in publishing this volume in a timely manner.

**—Dr. C. Jayachandran**
Professor of Marketing & International Business
Feliciano School of Business, Montclair State University
President, Academy of Global Business Research & Practice (AGBRP)

# *Preface*

Marketing is increasingly becoming a crucial aspect of organizational practice, as significant elements of marketing strategy are reflected in the structure, operations strategy, or customer service of most organizations, either for profit or not-for-profit. The healthcare sector is not exempt. Healthcare is essential in all societies, whether in developing or in developed countries, as the health sector is responsible for the preservation of health and well-being of a workforce; who are considered one of the most critical assets in an industrial economy. It is of concern that most institutions or practices in the health sector fare poorly in an assessment of customer value; in identifying market needs, and in providing adequate customer service which can stimulate continuance of patronage. In the health sector, customers are mostly seen as "patients" and not as "customers" who must be approached as of value and adequately paid attention to, so as to create/achieve customer satisfaction. A mere shift in thinking in the "patient" nomenclature will inspire a range of strategic responses and efficiencies that will influence how great the patient care experience in one practice can be clearly distinguished from others. Ironically, when healthcare marketing is discussed, it would appear that healthcare institutions that desire more clients, impliedly want more people to become unwell. The reality, however, is that as the most basic service needed worldwide, health management and marketing issues are intrinsically intertwined when quality and value are desired outcomes.

*Marketing in Healthcare-Related Industries,* pages xiii–xv
Copyright © 2020 by Information Age Publishing
All rights of reproduction in any form reserved.

In the 21st century, the healthcare service industry must, therefore, be seen through different lenses. Customer satisfaction and loyalty, strategic planning, and operational efficiency are amongst the critical success factors in both public and private health delivery systems. There is, therefore, the need for change in the way the sector operates. The organizational structure must be reviewed and redesigned to attract customers and develop a synergy between the target audience and the healthcare market.

The absence of these critical aspects of marketing healthcare industries has propelled this book for practitioners, but also for students at both undergraduate and postgraduate levels. *Marketing in Healthcare-Related Industries* is a practical book that is intentionally written with case studies to meet the needs of the 21st century in the healthcare market and to herald a pathway for the strategic development of the organizations in the healthcare industry. The book takes into cognizance the dynamics of the healthcare market in developing themes that will fill gaps, which healthcare industries have hitherto neglected in the marketing of their service to the desired target market.

The first chapter of the book introduces marketing healthcare by examining the history of marketing from a conceptual perspective. The subject of marketing has evolved over time, and the deliberate focus on its evolutionary phases allows the reader to carefully ascertain which marketing phase their healthcare institution currently operates in today. The second chapter discusses the seven Ps of the service marketing mix at the bedrock of healthcare, while the third chapter focuses on how society is evolving and how the outcomes for healthcare market development and the healthcare service industry can position themselves in relation to change. Most of the health industry activity around the world is carried out in the public sector, and consequently, Chapter 4 of the book focuses on how marketing can be used as a tool for improving the efficiency of public sector healthcare delivery.

Chapter 5 of the book highlights the importance of strategic planning in healthcare; Chapter 6 concentrates on innovation in healthcare delivery; Chapter 7 lays emphasis on stakeholder management in healthcare; and Chapter 8 directs our attention to understanding the behaviors of consumers to healthcare service encounters for proper positioning of healthcare service in a competitive market. Chapter 9 discusses manpower and people management, while Chapters 10, 11, and 12 provide insights into balancing healthcare service demand and effective relationship management to build loyalty in the healthcare service. These chapters also provide a tool kit to be used by practitioners and policymakers in the healthcare service, to improve their healthcare marketing efficacies.

The case studies in this book are fictional, with some based on real-life events. All names of persons and organizations have been changed or invented. These case studies are designed for classroom exercises only. The cases are not intended to reflect the state of customer service in the countries where we situated the events.

The book is a definitive resource for healthcare service marketing as it discusses the unique concepts and practices in the field. Case studies reinforce learning by drawing parallels to real-life experiences. Readers will gain valuable and actionable insights into effective healthcare service. The book is relevant to undergraduate and postgraduate students and also to healthcare practitioners.

# 1

# *An Introduction to Marketing in Healthcare*

## Chapter Outline

- Introduction
- The History of Marketing: The Five Concepts Defined
- Why Healthcare Marketing is Different
- Reasons for the Adoption of Healthcare Marketing
- Conclusion
- Review Questions
- Mini Case Study with Discussion Questions
- References

## Chapter Outcome

By the end of this chapter, the reader will be able to

- define healthcare,
- identify the importance of marketing in healthcare,
- describe the evolution of marketing,

*Marketing in Healthcare-Related Industries*, pages 1–23
Copyright © 2020 by Information Age Publishing
All rights of reproduction in any form reserved.

- discuss the peculiarities of healthcare marketing, and
- understand reasons that account for the adoption of marketing in the healthcare sector.

## Introduction

Healthcare is defined as efforts made, mainly by trained and licensed professionals, to maintain or restore physical, mental, or emotional well-being to a population. Healthcare systems are fast evolving in the 21st century. Due to technological advancements, as well as the growth of market-driven healthcare, competition, free enterprise, freedom of choice, patient empowerment, and an increasing number of patients becoming well informed, the healthcare space has also undergone significant changes over the years. It has, therefore, become crucial for firms in the healthcare space/medical practice to identify target markets, know the needs and wants of patients, and leverage marketing aggressively to create differentiated products and achieve profitability. The focus of marketing strategies in healthcare, as in every other service industry, should be customer satisfaction built through trust, dependability, and consistency in practice. Providers must maintain not only high clinical standards, but also provide services that create value and satisfy the patients.

Marketing is about identifying and meeting human and social needs (Kotler & Keller, 2012). Another acclaimed definition of marketing is that it is "the activity, set of institutions, and processes for creating, communicating, delivering, and exchanging offerings that have value for customers, clients, partners, and society at large" (American Marketing Association, 2013). From this definition, the consumer is the central focus of marketing. Within the healthcare sector, the consumer could be an individual patient, a physician, or other organizations that deal with health-related activities. Thus, patients should be the main focus of healthcare. The definition also highlights the essential activities under marketing, which result in customer satisfaction. In recent times, patient satisfaction has become a critical issue needed for the sustainability and growth of the healthcare industry.

Over the past few decades, marketing within the healthcare sector has advanced. Traditionally, marketing in the healthcare sector was viewed to be all about advertising. This represented a narrow outlook of marketing because advertising only, does not fully reflect and achieve the marketing tasks and aims of marketing. Marketing activities have become of paramount importance to healthcare providers, insurance companies, and other parties in trying to attract target consumers and satisfy consumers' healthcare needs.

Marketing helps provide an external perspective which brings added value to organizational planning. To attain success, it is essential for organizations to be responsive to the market, have the capacity to respond, have a clear vision of target, and have actionable steps. The marketing field has, in the past few decades, shifted attention beyond attracting customers and getting them to engage in a one-time transaction to focusing on retaining existing customers and getting them to be loyal to the firm and its brands. This approach, commonly known as relationship marketing, is aimed at building long-term relationships with customers. This change in focus presents useful implications for healthcare organizations in terms of structure and employees.

Over the years, the concept of marketing has been widely accepted. Irrespective of this acceptance, marketing of healthcare still faces several challenges. In years past, marketing was not considered as integral to the healthcare sector. As a result, the majority of healthcare administrators lack training in the business aspects of healthcare, and only a limited number of these administrators have obtained training or experience in marketing. However, for anyone involved in healthcare post the year 2000, the term marketing generates little emotional reaction, given the fact that the need for building strong hospital brands and the creation of superior customer experiences for patients is now commonplace. It is, however, noteworthy that three decades ago, healthcare marketing—as the concept is known today—was considered novel and controversial when first introduced to the industry 45 years ago. One of the pioneering hospitals to create formal positions for marketing staff is the Evanston Hospital in Evanston, Illinois, in 1975. Now, more than 40 years later, marketing has spread throughout healthcare into hospitals, group practices, rehabilitation facilities, outpatient care centers, and other healthcare organizations.

The idea of marketing is not new in most industries. However, in the healthcare sector, the narrative is different, as marketing is a relatively modern/recent phenomenon. Professionals in the healthcare sector that welcome marketing are concerned about the return on investment (ROI) that marketing can generate. At present, it appears healthcare organizations are seldom able to measure the cost of providing a specific service, thus, making a cost/benefit analysis extremely difficult.

The debate over the marketing budget of hospitals has been intense. The healthcare providers' immense rising interest in marketing comes at a time when many firms are shutting down facilities, tightening their belts, and some are laying off workers. The result is the belief that organizations' focus on consumer protection means that hospitals are spending considerable sums of money on marketing rather than focusing on patient care. The argument of the hospitals is that marketing is rather a strategic investment into the sustainable growth of the firms. Irrespective of the type of business, it can be argued today that marketing is still one of the essential requirements for an organization's success. The healthcare industry is becoming increasingly competitive, thereby stimulating marketing growth. Healthcare organizations, including hospitals, health systems, professional societies, and pharmaceutical companies need marketing to survive the competition and improve resilience and profitability. Lately, marketing has become even more important for pharmaceutical companies; they utilize a variety of marketing strategies to promote their products and educate people about diseases and treatment options.

Many in the healthcare business continue to be skeptical about the value of marketing to their businesses. For some health professionals, business practices still carry an unfavorable meaning that implies the suppression of clinical concerns to the bottom line. Some industry restrictions or regulations exist that pose as a bane to effective marketing in the healthcare sector. For example, many pharmaceutical companies are still hesitant to fully adopt social media, primarily due to lack of guidance.

This pessimism notwithstanding, primary care satellites, integrated delivery systems, managed care plans, and physician-hospital organizations are some of the elements that dominate the structure of the healthcare industry today (Berkowitz, 2010); and marketing excellence is needed to ensure all these components of the health industry work together seamlessly. Governments, employers, consumers, providers, and suppliers are all dealing with a new healthcare market that is increasingly customer-driven. This marketplace should be typified by a massive restructuring of the way healthcare organizations operate, and how healthcare service is purchased and delivered. To handle these forces of change, there is need for the implementation of effective marketing strategies if healthcare organizations want to remain competitive.

It has generally not been a problem for hospitals to generate income. However, medical expenses have skyrocketed. As a result, there is increasing pressure on healthcare providers to boost their revenues. The implication of this is that many of these firms are increasing their marketing budgets. In the United States, spending on healthcare marketing has increased sharply over the past two decades, rising from $17.7 billion in 1997 to $29.9 billion in 2016, with direct-to-consumer (DTC) advertising for prescription drugs and health services accounting for the most rapid growth, and pharmaceutical marketing to health professionals accounting for most promotional spending (Schwartz & Woloshin, 2019). In 2018, The Medical Marketing & Media Organization reported that the average marketing budget of healthcare companies in the United States recorded an additional growth of $2 million between 2017 and 2018 (Medical Marketing & Media Organization, 2019). This range cuts across independent hospitals to large healthcare systems with marketing budgets increasing as the size of the firm increases. Interestingly, the report made clear that although this budget may appear to be a lot of money, it only represented less than 1% of the typical hospital budget.

Similarly, pharmaceutical companies are adopting aggressive marketing strategies. In the United States, spending on DTC advertising increased from $1.3 billion in 1997 to $6 billion in 2016 (Schwartz & Woloshin, 2019). Large pharmaceutical companies spend more on marketing and sales than on research and development. For example, Johnson & Johnson alone spent $17.5 billion on sales and marketing in 2013, compared with $8.2 billion for R&D.

## The History of Marketing: A Conceptual Perspective

There are several definitions of marketing. The most widely accepted definition is from the American Marketing Association (2017), defines marketing as "the activity, set of institutions, and processes for creating, communicating, delivering, and exchanging offerings that have value for customers, clients, partners, and society at large."

The main aim of marketing is to respond to the needs and wants of consumers in the marketplace. This is exhibited in the development of a product that fits consumer needs or wants and the determination of the price of the product, which should be in line with the ability and willingness of customers to pay. Marketing also responds to consumer needs through the distribution of the product at the right place, which is convenient for the customer as well as creating awareness of the product, informing consumers about the benefits of the product and where to find it, and influencing them to buy more of the product through marketing communications. Hence, marketing must create value for customers through its activities.

Over the years, the philosophies that guide a firm's marketing efforts have been redefined. What should be the focus of firms when deploying a marketing strategy? A firm's marketing activities should be deliberately planned to focus on efficiency, effectiveness, and overall profitability. There are some key developments that have informed the formation of the marketing philosophy over several years. The concept of marketing has evolved through several developments, and the various phases in the evolution of the marketing concept are discussed next.

### The Production Concept

The time span for this concept extends roughly from the 1850s to the late 1920s. This concept suggests that consumers prefer products that are highly proliferated or available and cheap. Firms existent within this period were absorbed in achieving high efficiency in production, mass distribution, and highly reduced costs. The challenge with this concept, however, was that, firms were not interested in product specialization and were not keen on quality. The focus was on ensuring that products were available through multiple channels of distribution. Notably, there are hospitals at this stage in their own evolution. The production-oriented hospital would state, for instance, "Our basic function is to provide high-quality medicine. Accompanied by the highest forms of technology, we have physicians, nurses, and allied health personnel to provide this service, and we have administrators to keep the books" (Berkowitz, 2010, p. 12).

The product concept suggests that most individuals prefer products that give them the best quality, performance, or inventive or pioneering features. The challenge with this concept, however, was that managers were sometimes too confident in their products. Firms with this concept believed that a better product would automatically draw consumers to their shops. However, history has taught us that an innovative or enhanced product will only be successful if it is appropriately priced, distributed, advertised, and sold with the right segmentation and targeting strategies. An example of the product concept in healthcare would be hospitals who differentiate themselves from the competition by focusing on service quality and providing services that meet or exceed patient's needs and expectations. Oppong, Hinson, Adeola, Muritala, and Kosiba (2018) identified service quality as one of the major issues challenging healthcare organizations in Africa; improving service quality, therefore, can be a key differentiator for organizations in the continent.

### The Selling Concept

This concept suggests that consumers on their own will never buy enough of a firm's products. In the present day, the concept is often noticed when there is an unsought/unwanted commodity. In this instance, marketing strategies are aggressive (hard sell). An example of hard-sell practices is often seen with the sale of insurance. Firms are focused on merely selling what they produce rather than what the market may want. The effects of such aggressive strategies are that customers will complain and may not be interested in purchasing a firm's products any more.

For hospitals, the selling concept was most prominent when cost reimbursement became a common phenomenon in North America. Under cost-based reimbursement, hospitals were not focused on competing with other health institutions. Occupancy rates were high, and the length of time a patient stayed was not a problem. The cost involved in treating patients was not borne by the patients themselves but by third parties. At the sales stage in the healthcare industry, hospital administrators were focused on getting as many patients as possible. This was made possible by employing as many physicians as possible to attend to as many patients as the hospital could attract. The sales era preceded the times of utilization reviews. Primarily, the focus of hospitals was not on attracting efficient physicians who would care for patients in a limited period of time, but on attracting large numbers of physicians to meet demand.

The focus of a sales-oriented hospital could be captured thus: "We are a high-quality hospital providing numerous medical services to the market. We must attract physicians in the community who would want to admit to our facility. Moreover, we must encourage patients to want to come here" (Berkowitz, 2010, p. 13). The focus of the selling concept was based on the ability to sell. In consequence, the emphasis of hospitals in this era was to entice consumers of healthcare to patronize them. Some measures that were put in place to entice consumers to patronize certain hospitals included providing attractive lounges, introducing valet parking, building private clinics attached to the hospital facilities so that physicians could have the convenience of admitting patients to a hospital close to their consulting rooms for monitoring, among others.

## The Marketing Concept

The marketing concept emerged after the selling concept. The marketing concept was more customer-centric. The role of marketing was to bring the right buyers and businesses together in a near-perpetual, business-friendly, and customer-centered atmosphere. This concept suggests that the solution to realizing goals set by organizations is to be more effective in the creation, delivery, and communication of greater customer value to the target market. This would obviously have to be done better than competitors (Kotler & Keller, 2012). Selling is different from marketing; in selling, the emphasis is on the objectives of the seller. However, in marketing, the focus is on the buyer and what the buyer needs. In selling, the focus is on what the seller requires in order to convert an offering into money through a profitable exchange. However, in marketing, the central idea is to satisfy the needs of the consumer through a product that the consumer would see value in, in addition to the factors associated with the creation, delivery, and consumption of the offering. Many scholars have argued that firms that embrace the marketing concept have achieved greater performance (Kotler & Keller, 2012).

In healthcare, an institution that has embraced the marketing concept can be viewed as one that addresses the healthcare needs of the marketplace—a shift from a transactional focus to customer retention in the marketing paradigm. This marketing-oriented focus on the customer will lead to a product or service line that includes home healthcare, geriatric medicine, after-hour care, or wellness centers. The trend toward integrated delivery systems is to eliminate dealing with a fractionated healthcare system that consists of freestanding medical centers, providers, hospitals, and insurance firms. The formation of an integrated system enables healthcare organizations to deliver seamless healthcare services to buyers. The idea of integrated delivery systems is aimed at satisfying the customer through an organization that is responding to the demands of the customer effectively and efficiently.

---

### The Holistic Marketing Concept

The holistic marketing concept recognizes that everything that happens in marketing is important. Under this concept, activities within operations and marketing are significant. The entire firm's structure has the customer at the center, and firm-level activities revolve around this customer. At this level of marketing, the organization views marketing as a part of its corporate culture, and it is embedded at all levels of the organization. Hence, marketing is no longer the duty of the marketing department only, but of all functional areas of the organization. For instance, in the context of healthcare, the clinical nurse administrator markets a program on neurology. Similarly, the admitting desk staff and ward maintenance staff comprehend and appreciate the need to treat a customer right and maintain the hospital's customer orientation.

The holistic marketing concept is a unified concept that has guided several successful firms in the 21st century. Firms whose marketing activities begin and end with the customer do well. Under the holistic marketing concept, the development of patient-focused care in health organizations is achieved by establishing a marketing culture throughout the organization. The customer becomes the focus of these organizations, and all their activities are centered on the customer. To serve these customers better and offer convenience, hospitals cross-train employees to equip them with skills that will allow them to be as patient-responsible as possible. Aside from this, hospital admissions are accomplished on the floor where the patient is offered a bed. Also, rather than moving patients who need to use some hospital equipment to where the equipment is located, hospitals instead move the equipment, if possible, to where the patients are. Under holistic marketing, all healthcare employees understand the need to respond to consumer needs first.

Under the holistic marketing concept, the understanding of the customer increases, the value that the customer places in the firm improves, and ultimately, overall brand loyalty is enhanced. Concepts such as relationship management and customer delight are greatly emphasized in the holistic marketing concept.

## Why Healthcare Marketing is Different

The healthcare market is sharply dissimilar from the other types of service markets. This is even more the case when viewed from the customer's perspective. Health induces a sense of affinity between the customer and the providers and the need for involvement of the consumers. Serious health decisions sometimes have a small window of contemplation. Decisions need an amount of medical knowledge that some people may not possess. From a marketing standpoint, healthcare services are within the bracket of credence goods, which pose unique challenges compared to other consumer goods and services. These are types of goods with peculiar qualities that cannot be adequately judged or observed by the consumer following a purchase. This sometimes means that, healthcare customers occasionally find it difficult to judge the quality of the service they have received. To the extent that consumers lack the knowledge required to judge quality for themselves, they are quite vulnerable and rely on the opinions of the "expert" (healthcare provider) to appraise the quality of the clinical service they have received. In many cases, what the provider says is gospel.

The healthcare sector is unique. As such, the application of marketing philosophies and techniques in other contexts, cannot be transposed unto the field of healthcare. Therefore, unique marketing approaches that consider the unique characteristics of the healthcare sector is imperative. For example, patients, especially those with insurance, often do not know the price of the services consumed. However, several healthcare firms have sprung up across the globe. Competition among healthcare providers is getting intense (Corbin, Kelley, & Schwartz, 2001). Unlike many other services, healthcare has a direct bearing on the wellbeing of an individual (Gill & White, 2009). Effects of poor healthcare delivery cannot be compared to the post-purchase cognitive dissonance from having a bad haircut. The effects of purchase cognitive dissonance (i.e., post-purchase doubt about the wisdom of one's choice or one's experiences, feelings of post-purchase psychological tension, or anxiety) are more deep-seated and could have grave and fatal consequences in healthcare. For instance, a patient questions her judgment of choosing a local hospital for her cosmetic surgery: "Did I make the right choice? Should I have considered other hospitals?" These reactions have serious implications for the hospital as the uncertainty that has emerged from these reactions may transform into a dissatisfaction. Healthcare providers cannot just afford to view the provision of healthcare within the traditional commercial lenses. In the case of healthcare delivery, the customer undoubtedly must be at the center of every deed.

Another factor that also makes healthcare marketing unique and different is the nature of the demand for health services (Thomas, 2008). To some extent, demand for general healthcare services is elastic, and marketers can develop strategies to stimulate demand. However, major healthcare service encounters occur quite rarely and randomly. For instance, a critical occurrence as a heart attack or a stroke is likely to arise unexpectedly "and affect a small segment of the population. The marketing of such services represents a challenge for marketers who are faced with a disconnect between the service and the anticipated need" (Thomas, 2008, p. 7).

Additionally, the products offered in the healthcare sector are highly complex, and consumers may not easily understand them. For instance, it is difficult for a layperson to understand healthcare procedures, especially those that are technology-based, even upon explanations from health professionals. This inability to understand healthcare procedures can be attributed to the use of jargons or medical terms by health professionals, thereby making healthcare marketing so challenging.

Decision-making in healthcare is also delicate. On the one hand, information is critical. On the other hand, too much availability of the information can delay the decision-making process. Yet, in a completely different scenario, the evaluation of health analysis and information is becoming increasingly difficult for individuals who have very limited access to the information. In several countries in the developing world, access to the internet and low literacy rates are barriers to effectively accessing and assessing healthcare information. With the high perceived risk that could possibly come with a health-related choice, access to information that allows consumers the chance to rationally weigh the merits and demerits of a procedure or option is very critical. Not only does it have the potential to reduce the said perceived risk, but it can also psychologically invoke confidence in patients, as they are well empowered to make health-related decisions through access to detailed medical information. However, in cases where a decision must be made quickly, this becomes more critical, and the consumer may have to rely wholly on the caregiver. Additionally, as a result of technological advances, today's healthcare systems has provided new options in testing available procedures, further adding to the decision dilemma.

Traditionally, the healthcare provider controls all access to patient records and information, giving them sole responsibility in making healthcare decisions for patients. More recently, however, patients have desired to play a more active role in their receipt of healthcare services. This includes elderly patients who often opt for their healthcare information to be shared with a trusted family member to assist in the decision-making process. All that this proves is that control is important to the patient when it comes to their health (Wagner, Fleming, Mangold, & LaForge, 1994).

Another significant challenge faced in healthcare is the varying health insurance plans and healthcare systems across several countries. What is observed, however, is the increasing constraints of accessing doctors. As a result, this relationship built on trust that patients desire in a healthcare provider is becoming more challenging to create. In several cases, consumers deem making decisions regarding healthcare as particularly disturbing and one filled with unease for both the patients and their family. The need for information proves that consumers require help in comprehending the essential components of healthcare and the dynamic health needs over their lifetime. Current healthcare mediators may provide valued support; however, they appear as a rather poor auxiliary to a rapport with a principal and reliable family doctor. In discussing the price of services in healthcare, it appears to be chiefly ridiculous and annoying when viewed from the perspective of the consumer. Expensive bills are particularly problematic for the uninsured patient. Such patients are susceptible to the moods of the healthcare system.

In summary, the reason healthcare is different is because, as alluded to earlier, clinical quality is inflexibly viewed by patients as being paramount and tops all considerations. This perceived quality is even more accentuated when decisions to be made on a patient's health could be one that determines life and death. It is detrimental to a healthcare provider if quality clinical healthcare is viewed to have been compromised. A single incident of service failure in healthcare provision is enough to drive people away from the premises/facility. Consumers want to know that service providers did their best in any circumstance. They need strong assurances if they are to invest their lives into the hands of a healthcare provider. In cases where healthcare decisions may not even have dire consequences, consumers are not willing to accept low quality for cost-saving. Many would rather endeavor to comb the length and breadth of the communities and do anything humanly possible to secure the funds needed to receive the best healthcare. When an individual is ill, there is a sense of urgency that comes with it. This sense of urgency strongly affects patient decisions. Patients demand the quickest, most immediate, and effective handling of their ailment. However, despite this sense of urgency, especially in many parts of Africa, access to quality healthcare comes at a very high cost and medical services are woefully inadequate, with limited provision of government healthcare services. Several Africans risk their life savings since they do not have access to health insurance. Simply, healthcare is different from any other service when we bear in mind the complications and pressures that consumers face when making a decision that is related to their health.

The popular mantra "Your health is your wealth," reflects the paramount importance of healthcare. An individual who is well (where well-being encompasses mental and physical health) is usually happier and tends to enjoy a greater quality of life, that is, a person's overall satisfaction with life and self-perceptions of health. It could be argued that given the importance of health, healthcare providers will prioritize the delivery of superior service to patients. Increasing healthcare demand and increasing complexity of healthcare systems and procedures seem to have instead created significant challenges to healthcare institutions that seek to make their healthcare consumers (or patients) happy (Corbin et al., 2001). Healthcare marketing is most effective when information is appropriately communicated and channeled to the right audience. Health service marketing recognizes the immense value of marketing to generate awareness, encouraging repeat purchases, retention, and building customer lifetime value. Service marketing emphasizes customer satisfaction. Concepts such as customer delight and amazement have been advocated strongly within the service space. The focus is not on meeting needs, not even on exceeding them, but on completely amazing or dazzling the customer. However, an important question remains for service providers in the healthcare space which is: Why has one of the globe's most significant service industry, being the healthcare service, remained sluggish in recognizing or embracing the significance of service marketing principles in its totality? This is because the healthcare sector had previously not recognized the benefits of increased customer gratification and retention; of course, these are the sought outcomes of any fruitful marketing endeavor.

Service quality dimensions applicable to healthcare include factors such as completeness, consistency, and effectiveness. Consistency in healthcare service differs between producers, places, times, and customers. This heterogeneity is a result of the different professionals that administer healthcare services (e.g., physicians, nurses, etc.). This also demonstrates the factor of inseparability in healthcare services, where the service provider and the service rendered cannot be distinguished. In simpler terms, the output reflects the diverse skill sets of service providers. Healthcare professionals provide different outputs of services simply because educational background, specific skill sets, individual capabilities, and characters differ (Kay, 2007).

There are four distinguishing characteristics of healthcare services that distinguish them from pure physical goods. These are intangibility, heterogeneity, inseparability, and perishability. The intangibility of services, as mentioned earlier, is because they do not assume any physical form. Also, services usually cannot be adequately quantitatively evaluated, assessed, or systematically appraised before their consumption. As a result, the consumer's opinion of satisfaction is determined solely after purchase, where there can be post-purchase evaluation (Chahal & Mehta, 2013). Due to the presence of an attendant before a service can be provided and the corresponding personal communication that ensues, there is a high degree of variability in services. Services rely heavily on this personal communication between the service provider and the customer and this interaction even becomes a basis for judging the quality of the service. As a result of these characteristic irregularities in service outcomes, it can inhibit the provision of consistent and dependable service. These irregularities may even further hamper customer trust. In-service provision, the consumer, and the service provider cannot be separated. For example, a drug cannot be administered or surgery performed if the patient is not there. The physical presence of the patient is required before any of these can be done. This factors into the inseparability of services.

Additionally, the inseparability of services makes it impossible to disconnect the service from the provider. It further suggests that the production and consumption of service can take place concurrently. The last distinguishing factor of services is that they are perishable. This attribute of services makes it impossible to produce and stock services. Services as such cannot be inventoried. As a result of these features of services, it makes tracking of customer perceptions of quality difficult, more so within the healthcare sector.

With nearly every type of good, several evaluation approaches help to determine the offering that is the best fit for the particular customer. Consumers basically use three broad attributes to assess products or services—search, experience and credence criteria (Ford, Smith & Swasy, 1988). Under search criteria, evaluation properties are utilized in searching for the products. These factors may be determined and evaluated before the purchase of a commodity. Elements for evaluation include size and color. The next criterium is the experience properties—evaluation of these properties may be done during or after purchase. These include the liability, or ruggedness of a product.

The last criterion is the credence criteria. With this, it is nearly impossible to evaluate confidently even after a purchase has been made, and there has been consumption. An example that pertains to healthcare is the outcome of a major surgical procedure. When it comes to healthcare services, they have been characteristically low in their search properties, but rather high in the credence elements. In simpler terms, the patient in a healthcare facility is usually incapable of precisely choosing and assessing a physician before the patient and physician's encounter or interaction.

Further, patients in several cases are mostly incapable of recognizing and deeply understanding the outcomes of a patient and healthcare professional encounter. As such, there is much confidence in what the healthcare professional says (credence), as suggested earlier. Since patients are largely incapable of critically evaluating the available unique features of choice before purchase, the ability of service providers to assess the perception and utility of services is even more confounding.

The perception, evaluation, and utility of healthcare services are usually based on features that can be easily observed and comprehended by the patient, such as waiting time; the composure and civility of staff; how clean the rooms are; and the countenance of the nurse, doctor, technician, or other medical personnel. The overall appearance of the healthcare facility (physical evidence) is very critical to the evaluating consumer. In several cases, the features that a patient would use to judge the healthcare service would have very little to do with the service they sought and more to do with the seemingly "peripheral" elements of the facilities. Consumers need something to evaluate. Moreover, for them, the evaluation criteria would not be on the technical know-how since patients have minimal experience in judging that, but more to do with what they can see and touch when they walk into a facility to have an interaction with a caregiver.

The deployment of the marketing mix, tools that a marketer blends to successfully meet consumer needs profitably and create customer value, are obviously very weighty when it comes to healthcare marketing just as in any other marketing endeavor (Buccoliero, Bellio, Mazzola, & Solinas,

2016). The effects of marketing in the healthcare system are very significant. Branding a hospital as a specialized healthcare provider, for example, determines a swing in motivation for consumers. It equally determines the choice of executives, physicians, and other staff, all with the aim of delivering superior healthcare services that make the hospital function. A brand like this fundamentally changes the role of the said hospital within the community. When it comes to promotion, strategies bear on awareness and perceptions of health-related qualms and priorities. Marketing, therefore, plays an immensely crucial role in the healthcare system by linking healthcare services with their consumers and aids in the easy dispersal of information pertaining to patient health. In deploying healthcare marketing strategies, marketers need to understand this unique role marketing plays in healthcare delivery, as well as its ability to assist in boosting patient satisfaction and perceptions of healthcare service quality.

## Reasons for the Adoption of Healthcare Marketing

Healthcare is a fast-evolving industry. Marketing plays an important role in establishing a relationship between consumers and healthcare providers and satisfying their needs and wants. Now more than ever, it is critical for healthcare companies to market themselves, bearing in mind their target audience. A healthcare organization might design a marketing strategy around its major customer groups. The following justifications support the adoption of healthcare marketing today:

### Shared Vision of Market

A clear, shared vision of the market is crucial to healthcare organizational marketplace success, and the adoption of holistic marketing principles helps in achieving this marketplace success. To understand the marketplace, some relevant questions must be answered. These include: "Who are our organization's main customers and stakeholders?"; "What are the needs of these customers and stakeholders?"; and "What adjustment can the organization make in its marketing mix to meet the needs of this core target audience?" Also, it is important how the organization can differentiate itself from other providers.

### The Pressure to Be Market-Oriented

First, there is now a great pressure on healthcare organizations to become market-oriented, an approach that places significant focus on identifying the needs and desires of consumers and creating services that satisfy them. To achieve this, there must be a shared view that is accepted throughout the organization concerning the need for an improved marketing program. The pressure to be market-oriented should not be directed at senior management only, but at the organization in totality. All employees in the healthcare firm must have the strong urge to understand and respond to customer needs and wants. Healthcare marketing deals with identifying potential customers or market segments and their needs and wants. Information and reward systems must recognize that the value of customer orientation, and departmental program objectives as well as measurement systems must be tied to progress on this goal.

### Attracting Medical Staff and Employees

Two significant marketing concerns of organizations are the creation of customer loyalty and ensuring customer retention. Employees are recognized as a significant component, not only as an internal customer, but as a key link to long-term customer loyalty. As the healthcare industry expands, competition for skilled workers is increasing, and the demand for qualified healthcare professionals exceeds the supply. Many countries face a health workforce shortage, with the greatest burden borne by low-income countries, especially in sub-Saharan Africa and some parts of Asia. For example, Kenya is experiencing a health workforce shortage, particularly in specialized healthcare workers (Miseda, Were, Murianki, Mutuku, & Mutwiwa; 2017). Many health professionals are migrating from developing countries to developed countries. Hospitals and other healthcare providers are finding it necessary to promote themselves to potential employees by marketing the superior benefits that they offer to staff. In an era where the availability of various health professionals is limited, it has become vital for healthcare organizations to effectively market themselves to potential employees in order to attract them.

### Developing Respectable and Preferred Brands

Marketing in healthcare is not only for patients to search for physicians who can treat them, but even to look for job-seeking healthcare workers. The industry is fast evolving, and it is important that the industry adapts and keeps consumers well informed. In providing information, it must be timely and significant to ensure credibility. Marketing in healthcare must be carried out correctly, and consumers must be able to trust it. How well the practice is marketed tells how well providers understand their practice. In marketing, the consumer needs to be made aware of why a marketed practice is different from others and why it is the best in a host of other healthcare providers.

While branding in healthcare services is an emerging phenomenon, understanding the branding aspects of healthcare and its application and development strategies have become essential for healthcare firms "to identify comprehensively the dimensions, processes, and results of optimal branding in healthcare services and use them for planning, implementation, and management" (Khosravizadeh, Vatankhah, & Maleki, 2017). As a result of consumers being inundated with information as spoken about earlier, consumer power has increased. As such, in deciding which healthcare provider to deal with, for example in the case of hospitals, information such as the infection rate, the ranking of the hospital, and the number of specialists could influence consumers' opinions and selection. If hospitals do not consolidate their position, their competitors will consolidate theirs. This is achieved through word-of-mouth, and of course, by leveraging on the fact that consumers now have easy access to data. If a competitor's offering is all patients see, they will be more inclined to believe the competitor than they would a poorly marketed care provider (Padma, Rajendran, & Sai, 2009).

### *Developing an Integrated Communications Approach*

The healthcare space has also changed significantly. With the advent of healthcare facilities such as hospitals, pharmacies, surgery centers, and consumers who possess a strong sense of choice, the competition in the healthcare sector globally is very fierce. The rate at which consumers are also traveling outside their own country to receive medical care is also growing with countries like Thailand and India benefitting immensely from medical tourism. This is also evidently seen in the health services of hospitals accredited by the U.S.-based Joint Commission International (JCI), and have become one of the main drivers in the growth of medical tourism (PBB, 2019) . Since marketing in healthcare has also become more intricate and versatile, there is a need for a more unified promotional and communication approach. The traditional use of billboards, print media, or even high-quality television campaigns no longer cut it. There is a need for more engagement and not shoving messages down the throats of consumers. Social media platforms are actively being used to position the brands of healthcare companies; an attractive website is crucial in healthcare marketing, using video to provide information and even develop seminars for prospects to make a choice and also learn more about the healthcare services of the company. The fast-changing technological landscape makes it more necessary for healthcare brands to be at the cutting edge of leveraging technology, not only in the clinical practice, but in marketing efforts as well. Now, the consumer is not only interested in paying for great services, but is also interested in buying from a good brand. Some hospitals sponsor free lectures from renowned experts or provide virtual tours of their facility. The use of humor in advertising campaigns is increasing in healthcare, letting go of "hard to digest" advertisements and leveraging humor appeal (Limbu & Huhmann, 2012).

### Delivering Service Quality

Quality determination in healthcare is subjective and based on the process undertaken in administering the service, as well as the interaction between the service provider and the customer (Ramsaran, 2008). As a result, the five service quality (SERVQUAL) dimensions of "reliability, responsiveness, assurance, empathy, and tangibles" (Parasuraman, Zeithmal, & Berry, 1988, p. 12) are also applicable in the healthcare service. Among them, reliability and responsiveness are critical factors that impact patients' satisfaction with hospitals (Meesala & Paul, 2018). Within each of these dimensions would be a level of tolerance that a patient possesses in relation to the delivery of healthcare. From the viewpoint of service delivery, it is important that healthcare providers comprehend these tolerance levels associated with the various dimensions of service quality (Rooma, 2008). There is increased competition between healthcare providers for the consumer/patient, which places pressure on healthcare organizations to deliver healthcare efficiently. Additionally, with the significant evolution of healthcare practice into a service sector, patients are now being considered as customers. As a result, they are up in arms across the globe expecting better service. Consequently, easy access to healthcare professionals, convenience, and in some cases, luxury health services, are now very significant elements that altogether add to the patient's assessment of the quality of healthcare that they have received.

### Informing and Educating Consumers

Healthcare consumers are becoming increasingly involved in making healthcare choices and in expressing expectations and opinions about different treatment options. They are increasingly seeking health and healthcare service information, primarily via the Internet. Thus, advertising and other marketing communications about healthcare alternatives for consumers are not only desirable, but necessary if people are to make informed decisions from among many options. As greater consumer access to healthcare information could improve patient decision-making, healthcare organizations need to better utilize marketing tools to inform consumers about the kinds and levels of services to be offered in order to assist their healthcare decisions (Kay, 2007).

## Conclusion

The world economy has experienced tremendous growth in the healthcare sector. To adequately satisfy customers/patients, there is now an increasing need to implement marketing strategies and concepts in healthcare. The fact remains that healthcare providers who expertly craft their strategies with marketing concepts will end up providing better customer-driven healthcare than their competitors.

Marketing in healthcare has transitioned from being viewed as just advertising to the all-inclusive approach of adequately satisfying patient needs (Wagner et al., 1994), which, of course, embodies what marketing is about, basically. Consumers (patients) are educating themselves now by constantly acquiring information from several sources and expecting that their needs will be met, not only in terms of the provision of clinical needs, but that their technical and functional requirements will also be achieved in service provision parameters. Consumers are currently evaluating their satisfaction in healthcare provision with their entire service experience. As a result, healthcare practices must embrace this change in consumer (patient) behavior and deliver the desired customer service. As with every service encounter, consistently satisfied customers transition to becoming loyal customers. They, as such, become lucrative contributors to the progress of their healthcare service as well as the entire function of their selected service provider through positive feedback expressed through positive word-of-mouth. Satisfied customers are loyal to their caregivers and non-passive contributors to the result of their health. Generally, in in-services, be it the conventional selling concept or the intricate patient and physician relationship, there are philosophies and areas of service critical to the creation of customer utility and the establishment of brand loyalty (Moliner, 2009). The intricacies and peculiarities related to service delivery in the sector require a systematic appraisal, benchmarking, and tracking systems, which are very significant in the determination of the patient utility that is being sought.

The medical landscape is a fast-evolving one. There is an increased need for healthcare companies to push their offerings. The times are changing within the healthcare sector and there are calls for healthcare organizations to transition into market-oriented institutions. Irrespective of this call, several hospitals and other medical groups find the transition challenging. This is because, over the years, healthcare organizations have not fully understood the concept of being market-driven, that is, firms' policy or strategy guided by market trends and customer needs, as well as the benefits derived from marketing. Marketing success can be achieved within the healthcare organization when the institution has enough staff who have obtained training and experience in marketing as well as devoted to improving the organization's efforts in relation to marketing. Hence, employees of healthcare institutions must be open-minded to marketing ideas.

The domain of healthcare marketing is not only about creating a very informative website, using billboards, or even pushing out flyers; it encompasses a provider's ability to build excellent relationships, ensure the satisfaction of patients and referrers, fully understand their target market, and overall, deploy the marketing mix in an optimum way. The success of a marketing strategy should be measured on a significant return on investment. If current strategies are not yielding this, then there is a need to restructure the marketing campaign.

Finally, for a healthcare provider's practice to see growth, they must deploy a marketing strategy that is effective and can draw new consumers, successfully keep old patients and excellent staff and also sustain existing relationships with other referrers. Significant time must be devoted to improving marketing efforts to developing an understanding of how these efforts integrate with other organizational priorities. The organization must, therefore, develop a clear set of actionable tactics to respond to market needs.

## Review Questions

1. Define marketing and explain the evolution of the marketing concept with key examples.
2. Briefly elaborate on the importance of marketing and how it can be applied to healthcare.
3. Explain why there is presently a need for the implementation of marketing strategies in the healthcare industry.
4. With a key focus on this assertion, describe why healthcare marketing differs from the marketing of other products.

## MINI CASE-STUDY: IMPROVING CUSTOMER SERVICE EXPERIENCE AT PEACE HOSPITAL

Helen Duke was recently promoted to the position of Assistant Head of Nursing in Peace Hospital, Lagos, Nigeria. Her new position came with some administrative roles, which included ensuring improved customer service experience. She had been with the hospital for eight years as a Registered Nurse and witnessed the deplorable state of the hospital's physical environment. She often gets frustrated at the sight of the hospital's physical environment as it does not correspond to the quality of care delivered by its employees, who were undoubtedly committed to the welfare of the patients. With her new role, Helen felt she could make a difference.

She discovered many things were wrong with the physical environment ranging from leaking roofs, damaged furniture in the waiting areas, falling ceilings, too old and dilapidated beds in the wards, inadequate supply of water, noise-making generator, and untidy parking areas, amongst others. Helen thought within herself that if the degree of attention and care given to patients corresponds with the attention paid to the physical environment, Peace Hospital would have created a top of mind awareness (TOMA) among its existing customers as well as potential clients. She understood the importance of improvement of the servicescape to the general impression visitors formed of the hospital. The servicescape refers to the physical environment wherein the service is carried out; the physical surroundings often influence the behaviours of customers and employees in service organizations.

First, she had to start with the appearance of the nurses. When Helen was newly employed, she was disgusted by the dress sense of the employees. They dressed in such a way that patients, visitors and even the employees were confused about who is who and who does what. She immediately enforced a policy that assigned uniform colours to associated employees according to their various departments. Therefore, there was ease of identification, which also inculcated professionalism in their appearance. Secondly, she tried to reduce the noise level. Her efforts in this regard significantly enhanced the environment for both patients and staff members.

Regarding the improvement needed in the physical environment, Helen decided to draw up a plan to be proposed to the Chief Medical Director (CMD) of Peace Hospital, knowing well that her ideas will make the hospital more marketable. She was notified of the likely rejection of her proposal by the CMD due to the costs that will be involved. Notwithstanding, she insisted that at worst-case scenario, the hospital could call for volunteers who would contribute to improving the hospital's facility and Peace

Hospital will be the hospital it should be, where excellent health care delivery matches with the servicescape.

### Questions

1. Helen was very keen on ensuring that the servicescape corresponds with the quality of care provided at Peace Hospital. Do you think that was necessary? What role does improving servicescape play in marketing Peace Hospital?
2. Assuming the CMD rejects Helen's plan, how would you go about it if you were in Helen's shoes?
3. Discuss key factors to put into consideration in delivering quality service in healthcare

## References

American Marketing Association. (2017). *Definition of marketing.* Retrieved from https://www.ama.org/the-definition-of-marketing-what-is-marketing/

Berkowitz, E. N. (2010). *Essentials of health care marketing.* (3rd ed.). Ontario, Canada: Jones & Bartlett.

Buccoliero, L., Bellio, E., Mazzola, M., & Solinas, E. (2016). A marketing perspective to "delight" the "patient 2.0": New and challenging expectations for the healthcare provider. *BMC Health Services Research, 16,* 47.

Chahal, H., & Mehta, S. (2013). Modeling patient satisfaction construct in the Indian healthcare context. *International Journal of Pharmaceutical and Healthcare Marketing, 7*(1), 75–92.

Corbin, C. L., Kelley, S. W., & Schwartz, R. W. (2001). Concepts in service marketing for healthcare professionals. *The American Journal of Surgery, 181*(1), 1–7.

Ford, G. T., Smith, D. B., & Swasy, J. L. (1988). An empirical test of the search, experience and credence attributes framework. In M. J. Houston (Ed.), *NA—Advances in consumer research* (Vol. 15; pp. 239–244).Provo, UT: Association for Consumer Research.

Gill, L. G., & White, L. (2009). A critical review of patient satisfaction. *Leadership in Health Services, 21*(1), 8–19.

Kay, M. J. (2007). Healthcare marketing: What is salient? *International Journal of Pharmaceutical and Healthcare Marketing, 1*(3), 247–363.

Khosravizadeh, O., Vatankhah, S., & Maleki, M. A. (2017). Systematic review of medical service branding: Essential approach to hospital sector. *Annals of Tropical Medicine and Public Health, 10*(5), 1137–1146.

Kotler, P., & Keller, K. L. (2012). *Marketing management.* Upper Saddle River, NJ: Pearson.

Limbu, Y. B., & Huhmann, B. (2012). An examination of humor and endorser effects on consumers' responses to direct-to-consumer advertising: The moderating role of product involvement. *International Journal of Pharmaceutical and Healthcare Marketing, 6*(1), 23–38.

Medical Marketing & Media. (2019, March 4). *Average marketing budgets of health care companies in the United States in 2017 and 2018, by type (in million U.S. dollars)* [Chart]. Retrieved from https://www.statista.com/statistics/275384/marketing-budgets-of-us-health-care-companies/

Meesala, A., & Paul, J. (2018). Service quality, consumer satisfaction and loyalty in hospitals: Thinking for the future. *Journal of Retailing and Consumer Services, 40*, 261–269.

Miseda, M. H., Were, S. O., Murianki, C. A., Mutuku, M. P., & Mutwiwa, S. N. (2017). The implication of the shortage of health workforce specialists on universal health coverage in Kenya. *Human resources for health, 15*(1), 80. https://doi.org/10.1186/s12960-017-0253-9

Moliner, M. A. (2009). Loyalty, perceived value and relationship quality in healthcare services. *Journal of Service Management, 20*(1), 76–97.

Oppong, E., Hinson, R. E., Adeola, O., Muritala, O., & Kosiba, J. P. (2018). The effect of mobile health service quality on user satisfaction and continual usage. *Total Quality Management & Business Excellence.* https://doi.org/10.1080/14783363.2018.1541734

Padma, P., Rajendran, C., & Sai, L. P. (2009). A conceptual framework of service quality in healthcare: Perspectives of Indian patients and their attendants. *Benchmarking: An International Journal, 16*(2), 157–191.

Parasuraman, A., Zeithmal, V. A., & Berry, L. (1988). A multiple-item scale for measuring consumer perceptions of service quality. *Journal of Retailing, 64*(1), 12–40.

PBB Patients Beyond Borders. (2019). *Medical tourism and statistics.* Retrieved from https://www.patientsbeyondborders.com

Ramsaran, R. (2008). The relative importance of service in dimensions in a healthcare setting. *International Journal of Healthcare Quality Assurance, 21*(1), 104–124.

Rooma, R. R.-F. (2008). The relative importance of service dimensions in a healthcare setting. *International Journal of Healthcare Quality Assurance, 21*(1), 104–124.

Schwartz, L. M., & Woloshin, S. (2019). Medical marketing in the United States, 1997–2016. *JAMA, 321*(1), 80–96.

Thomas, R. K. (2008). Health services marketing: a practitioner's guide. New York, NY: Springer Science & Business Media.

Wagner, H. C., Fleming, D., Mangold, W., & LaForge, R. (1994). Relationship marketing in healthcare. *Marketing Health Services, 14*(4), 42–47.

# 2

# Services Marketing as the Bedrock of Healthcare Marketing

## Chapter Outline

- Introduction
- Evolution of the Services Marketing Concept: From 4Ps to 7Ps
- Challenges of Cost-Based Pricing
- Challenges of Competition-Based Pricing
- Challenges of Demand-Based Pricing
- Services in the Modern Economy
- The Importance of Differences Among Services
- The Importance of Marketing Healthcare Services
- Integrating Marketing With Other Functions in Healthcare Organization
- Conclusion
- Review Questions
- Mini Case Study With Discussion Questions
- References

*Marketing in Healthcare-Related Industries,* pages 25–43
Copyright © 2020 by Information Age Publishing

## Chapter Outcome

By the end of this chapter, the reader will be able to

- explain what services marketing is,
- discuss the evolution of services marketing concept from 4Ps to 7Ps,
- discuss the growth of the service sector globally,
- explain how services are dominating the modern economy,
- discuss the importance of differences among services, and
- discuss how services pose distinctive marketing challenges.

## Introduction

All trade and commercial activities are categorized under three headings, namely: primary, secondary, and tertiary. The primary activities of an economy include, but are not limited to, agriculture, fishing, forestry, and mining. On the other hand, the secondary and tertiary activities include manufacturing, processing, construction, distribution, and services. Soriya and Dhaigude (2016) describe the service sector as an aspect of the economy that produces intangible goods. The authors explain that the end results of the productions of the service sector are products that cannot be held nor touched and the activities in the service sector cover: retail, hotels, banks, real estate, health, education, social work, recreation, computer services, media, communications, gas, electricity, and water supply. Over the years, the service sector has emerged as the most dynamic sector of the world economy, contributing half of the world's gross value added, half of the world's employment, one fifth of global trade, and more than half of the world's direct investment flows.

Over the years, service has been variously defined by different scholars and organizations. The numerous attempts by these scholars and bodies to come out with a definition of what service is, emphasize that there is no one best and generally accepted definition of the subject matter—service. Philip Kotler (2002) conceptualizes service as any activity which is performed by one party to another, which is mainly intangible and does not lead to the ownership of anything. He adds that the production of a service may not be tied to a physical product. Zeithaml and Bitner (2000) also argue that services are "deeds, processes and performance." Baruch, Quin, Penny, and Paquette (1987) equally provide a compelling description of what a service is by equating the subject matter to all commercial activities whose output is not a physical product or construction, but one which is generally consumed at the time of its production, and one that provides added value in forms such as convenience and amusement, among others. Furthermore, Baruch et al. (1987) posit that the unique intangibility feature of a service is of concern to its first purchaser.

Recently, services are widely being accepted as the medium through which organizations meet and engage with their target and their potential markets (Irons, 1997; Strydom, 2005). Research shows that inventive organizations that are known to offer novel services, as well as inimitable and matchless customer services, are currently succeeding in markets where established organizations have failed (Lovelock, Patterson & Walker, 1998; Strydom, 2005). What this means is that for business organizations and practitioners to survive in today's globally competitive and information-rich world, a marketing strategy that seeks to provide stupendous service quality and outstanding and memorable customer experience needs to be carefully crafted and implemented. Fortunately, a search through some literature shows that business organizations are competing strategically through service quality for greater differentiation in today's competitive marketplace.

This chapter introduces service marketing and discusses it extensively, laying a foundation before applying it to the healthcare setting.

## Evolution of the Services Marketing Concept: From 4Ps to 7Ps

The subject of the evolution of the marketing mix concept continues to receive massive attention from scholars and practitioners. Extant research traces the origin of the marketing mix, better known as the four Ps (4Ps), to the late 1940s where Professor James Culliton, a professor of marketing at the Harvard University, was credited to be the first to mention a mix in an article entitled, "The Management of Marketing Costs" (Dominici, 2009). Since then, the marketing mix concept has become a widely used term since the phrase was coined by Neil Borden during his American Marketing Association presidential speech in 1953 (Van Waterschoot & Van den Bulte, 1992). The Marketing Mix, known as the 4Ps, which are product, price, place, and promotion, have been developed tactically to create and exceed customer satisfaction. Over the years, the concept has received some criticisms for its focus on fast-moving consumer goods (FMCG; Kent, 1986; Gronroos, 1994).

According to some scholarly studies, the growth of service industries coupled with the unique characteristics of services has shown that the traditional 4Ps were not fully adequate in the context of service marketing. In order to rectify this shortfall in the traditional marketing mix, the seven Ps (7Ps) were created (Booms & Bitner, 1981). More specifically, the 7Ps was developed in an attempt to solve the problems associated with the marketing of intangible services. The extended marketing mix preserved the traditional 4Ps and added three additional elements. The three other Ps include: physical evidence, process, and people (Vargo & Lusch, 2008); these will be discussed in the subsequent paragraphs. Figure 2.1 shows key attributes of the marketing mix.

## Product

The first element in the marketing mix is the product. A product is anything, including goods, services, or ideas that can be offered to a market for attraction, acquisition, or use to satisfy a want or need (Kotler, 2000). For a product to be successful on the market, the marketers need to take some factors into consideration in its design, production, and marketing. These factors include, but are not limited to, the product benefits, features, quality, packaging, branding, and warranties. In healthcare, a product mainly represents inpatient and outpatient services provided by healthcare providers.

## Price

Price can be said to be the value placed on a product or the amount of money that is charged for something considered of value. It is actually what the customer should give up in order to obtain benefits offered by the marketer's product. All things being equal, the marketer would wish for the highest possible price, and the consumer would also wish for the lowest possible price. In this regard, there is a need for a careful balance to ensure that prices fixed for the product are affordable to the consumer while enabling the marketers to make some profit.

### Pricing Services

Due to the peculiar characteristics of services, pricing is a challenging task. Healthcare pricing is complex and varies across geographic boundaries. There is a lack of price transparency in healthcare, which is assumed to be one of the main drivers of rising healthcare cost. Rising healthcare cost has been one of the major concerns for patients, especially those without comprehensive health insurance coverage. Therefore, there is a call for greater price transparency and a reduction in health premiums and

| People | Product | Price | Promotion | Physical Evidence | Processes | Place |
|---|---|---|---|---|---|---|
| Those involved in service delivery, their behavior, attitudes, and interactions | Quality, features, options, style, brand name, packaging, services | Listed price, discounts, allowances, payment period, credit | Advertising, selling, sales promotion, publicity, public relations | Information in leaflets, components facilitating the performance and communication of the service | Viewed as a system of inputs and outputs (e.g., information, people); mechanisms involved in the delivery of a product or service; policies and procedures | Distribution channels, coverage, location, convenience, availability |
| *Stakeholders* | *The Service* — Features, location, design, branding | *Financial Management* — Tendering contracts | *Vision, Values, Culture* — Branding, design of literature, letterheads, leaflets | *Prospectus* — Website, newsletters, organization's facilities and buildings | *Surveys* — Evaluation of surveys, complaints procedure, quality management, consultation, charter mark, investors in people, open door policy | *The Organization* — Where situated, opening times |

**Figure 2.1** Key attributes of the marketing mix. *Source:* Booms & Bitner, 1981.

out-of-pocket expenses. Some pharmaceutical companies have been criticized for charging an excessive or inappropriate price for branded drugs. Monetary pricing is not the only price relevant to the service customer; nonmonetary costs represent other sources of sacrifices when buying and using a service; these include

- time costs,
- search costs,
- convenience costs, and
- psychological costs.

### Pricing Strategies

Service firms use three main pricing strategies, including costs-based, competition-based, and demand-based pricing. All these pricing strategies, however, have their own peculiar problems that need to be taken into consideration.

### Challenges of Costs Based Pricing

Cost is difficult to trace or calculate in service businesses, particularly where a firm provides multiple services. If you were a restaurant owner, you could charge people only for the food you are serving. However, then who will pay for the lovely ambience you have created for your customers? Who will bear the cost of the musical band playing? An analysis of these elements will lead to effective costing. Commonly, in pricing a service, factors such as labor, material cost, and overhead costs, are considered. By adding a profit markup, you get your final service pricing. Employee time rather than materials are challenging to estimate. The actual service cost may under-represent the value of the service to the consumer.

**Challenges of competition-based pricing.** This approach focuses on prices charged by other industry players within the same service categories. Smaller firms may charge too little and not make enough to remain in business. The heterogeneity of services across and within service providers makes this approach complicated.

**Challenges of Demand-Based Pricing.** The first two approaches to pricing are based on the company and its competitors rather than on customers. This approach, however, focuses on what customers will pay for the services provided. Challenges with this approach can arise when services require time, inconvenience, and psychological search costs for which the monetary price must be adjusted to compensate and vice-versa. This is especially challenging because companies must determine the value that customers will pay for each nonmonetary aspect involved in the service.

In healthcare, pricing is complex, which should take into account many different factors. Thus, healthcare organizations use various pricing strategies. Cost-plus pricing in which the selling price is determined by adding a markup to the cost of goods and services is a common pricing strategy among private hospitals. Fee-for-service (FFS), where physicians and healthcare providers are paid based on the number of services provided, is a popular payment method in the United States (Berenson & Rich, 2010). On the other hand, patients and payers may benefit from a bundled pricing strategy in which a single payment is made to providers for all services performed to treat a patient undergoing a specific episode of care, as it may promote price transparency and help to curb healthcare costs. In order to control the cost of care, managed care organizations use capitation payments in which healthcare providers are paid a fixed monthly fee based on the number of enrollees. In the United States, pharmaceutical and health insurance companies have become oligopolistic markets; they generally do not engage in price competition.

## Place

Place refers to where the service product is going to be located. For instance, the best place to open up a petrol station is on the highway or in the city as opposed to a place where there is minimum traffic. In the same vein, the most appropriate location for a software company is a business hub, which has several other companies nearby rather than in a town or a rural area. It is of great importance that the distribution outlets are strategically located to make it very convenient for customers and other members to do business. In healthcare, examples of the place component of the marketing mix would be the locations of healthcare facilities, opening hours, and appointment types (e.g., walk-in or same day). Changes in the healthcare service delivery system have resulted in a decline in hospital inpatient days and a growth in ambulatory services. Interestingly, as a response to the changing economic incentives within the healthcare delivery system, numerous types of outpatient services have emerged, and also, a variety of locations for the delivery of services have developed.

## Promotion

In the views of marketers, promotion (marketing communications) is a significant aspect of the marketing mix. Service firms rely on promotion to communicate positioning to customers. As such, promotions have become critical in the marketing of services. It adds tangibility, which allows the consumer to evaluate the service offering. The promotional mix, otherwise known as the marketing communication mix, entails six elements: (a) advertising, (b) public relations, (c) sales promotion, (d) personal selling, (e) direct mail, and (f) word-of-mouth. Advertising is an impersonal communication used by service firms to add to the customer's knowledge of the service, persuade the customer to buy, and differentiate the service from that of competitors. For the marketing of services to be successful, tenacious advertising must be ensured, and service firms usually must spend a considerable sum on advertising. Since the core product is intangible, service marketers find promotional aspects difficult. They choose the tangible elements that come along with the product for promotion. Airlines, for example, promote their service by advertising about the quality of their cuisine, the width and pitch of the seats, and the quality of their in-flight service. Nowadays, advertising is also extensively undertaken for financial services, telecommunication, retailing, and so on. Hospitals, insurance firms, and pharmaceutical companies are increasingly transitioning from push to pull marketing strategies and promoting their products and services directly to consumers through mass media. The Internet has become an invaluable communication tool for healthcare service marketers. Social media usage by healthcare organizations has increased dramatically; about 95% of the top-ranked hospitals use social media (Smith, 2017). Pharmaceutical companies historically relied on personal selling, sales promotion, and medical journal advertising, but in recent years, they are increasingly employing a pull strategy and promoting prescription drugs directly to consumers.

### People

In all organizations, people play a decisive role. Employees working in service organizations such as banks, hotels, and salons are the frontline contact people with the customers. The role of these frontline people decides the success of the service organization. According to Berry and Parasuraman (2004), a service organization can only be as good as its people. The strength and success of the service organization lie in the quality of the service personnel working in the organization. The behavior and attitude that service personnel exhibit, influences the customer's overall perception of the quality of the service delivered.

For instance, the behavior and attitude of a restaurant waiter determine whether the customer will patronize the services of that restaurant both at that moment and later. For this reason, it is necessary for service organizations to attract, develop, motivate, and retain qualified employees for the best customer service. People working in the service organizations are viewed as "the first level of customers." Employees who receive good training and are well motivated in terms of remuneration and other benefits, tend to render the best services to customers. This is why internal marketing is a crucial activity in shaping the "people" element of the service marketing mix. The purpose of internal marketing is to instill the sense of responsibility, responsiveness, and unity of purpose among service employees. It removes functional barriers to organizational effectiveness. Internal marketing involves the development of customer orientation and the alignment of internal and external marketing, to ensure effective relationship marketing.

Aside from sales personnel possessing the capacity to influence customer's perception of the service offering, customers can also do so through word-of-mouth. Customers who are satisfied with the service of a service provider will, in turn, tell others about their experiences. Some of the people these customers talk to are also likely to try the services of the organization in question. The majority of the customers of service firms decided to transact business with the firms because of recommendations from relatives, friends, and colleagues, among others. At the same time, a dissatisfied customer may talk ill of the service he/she had received, so the service provider must ensure total satisfaction of the existing customers.

## Physical Evidence

Another relevant element in the marketing mix of services is physical evidence. Physical evidence is crucial in the service context, considering the intangibility of services. Customers of service firms often seek signals to enable them to evaluate or predict the outcome of the service to be rendered. Mitchell and Greatorex (1993) identified that physical evidence and memory generally serve as the only source of evidence-based information on which service consumers make purchasing decisions. Physical evidence enables service organizations to describe the service-product and highlight their distinctive qualities. The physical evidence of service providers covers the facilities, objects, communication, and so on.

Physical evidence has two components: peripheral evidence and essential evidence. Peripheral evidence does not deliver independent value to the customer, yet can be possessed by the consumer. For instance, a bank's checkbook given to the customer is on its own of no value to the customer unless he or she has sufficient money in the account. Though peripheral, evidence has little independent value, they are the real source of competitive differentiation. They do have an impact on customer perception about the nature of service. Essential evidence cannot be possessed by the consumer; however, essential evidence forms a dominant part of the services and have independent value to the customers. Examples of essential physical evidence include the ambience of a university campus, a bank, a car, an aircraft, a hotel building, and the likes. Both peripheral evidence and essential evidence are needed for successful service delivery and customer satisfaction. Therefore, they need to be effectively coordinated. For instance, to satisfy customers and enhance the image of an airline, the service provider will have to coordinate the aircraft (essential evidence) and the food, the uniform of the cabin crew, beverages, and souvenirs, among others (peripheral evidence).

### *Process*

In the service context, the service creation and delivery process are of utmost importance. This is because customers often do not differentiate the service delivery system from the service itself. The success of service marketing is, thus, dependent on the decisions made concerning the processes involved in service delivery. Processes, in the service context, relate to tasks, schedules, routines, procedures, activities, and mechanisms through which a service is delivered to a customer. For example, services organizations such as hospitals and educational institutions deliver services by adopting procedures that allow for smooth delivery of services. When a type of service is occasional and rarely repeated, intermittent operations are suitable. For example, service organizations offering consultancy and advertising adopt varied (sporadic) operations to suit the needs of their clients.

## Services in the Modern Economy

As the economies of nations improve, the economic activities tend to move from primary activities, where the majority of economic activities are undertaken using very high human effort to other more secondary options. There are three main stages to a nation's economic development. These are the pre-industrial society, the industrial society, and the post-industrial society.

### *Pre-industrial Society*

At this stage, economic activities are mostly for the production of primary commodities or raw materials using human efforts. These activities are also at the mercy of the weather and other elements such as soil quality and availability of water. They are also characterized by low productivity and high unemployment. At this stage, the majority of people do not pay others for services, but undertake these activities by themselves.

## Industrial Society

This stage is characterized by the production of goods as the main activity. There is much mechanization and increased standards of living, where the quality of living is measured by the availability of goods. At this stage, the affluent in the society do engage the services of others for many of the routine activities they used to do by themselves. This results in some demand for service companies.

## Post-Industrial Society

In a post-industrial society, there is further improvement upon the standards of living. The quality of life is measured by the quality of health, education, and recreation shared by members of such a society. The service sector is the wheel through which such an economy thrives. Globalization, with its associated risks and benefits, is credited with the way societies across the globe are moving rapidly from industrial to the post-industrial society. The economy in the post-industrial society is much more dependent on the service industry. It is, therefore, important for these service delivery companies to undertake effective service marketing to gain a preferential advantage over their competitors. Interestingly, as the economic circumstance of humans improves, their need for services also increases, as can be illustrated with Abraham Maslow's hierarchy of needs. Maslow's hierarchy of needs is a motivational theory in psychology that explains the nature of human needs and what urges people to want to satisfy a certain need at a particular point in time. The theory consists of a five-tier model of human needs. These human needs are often depicted as hierarchical levels within a pyramid. According to the needs theory, human needs can be classified into five levels, starting from the bottom of the hierarchy to the top, the needs are physiological as are safety, love and belonging, self-esteem, and self-actualization. Maslow's hierarchy of needs theory holds that the needs depicted at the bottom of the hierarchy or the pyramid must be satisfied before individuals can attend to needs higher up the hierarchy. Consequently, an individual often needs to fulfil his/her basic needs such as food, shelter, clothing, and other survival needs before considering fulfilling safety needs, esteem needs, and the others, as illustrated in Figure 2.2.

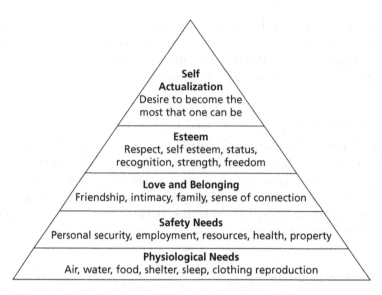

**Figure 2.2**   Maslow's Hierarchy of Needs. *Source:* McLeod, 2018.

Over the years, the activities of service firms and service organizations have become the mainstay of the world economy. By their provisions, service firms are increasingly dominating the expanding world economy by offering new services that satisfy existing customer needs and preferences that consumers initially did not know they needed. For instance, nearly five decades ago, when the first electronic file sharing system was created, it is likely that the future demand for online banking, website hosting, or email providers was not anticipated. These days, online banking and similar file-sharing activities have become the order of the day. To most people, they cannot live without these IT services in their day-to-day activities.

Interestingly, today, similar revolutions are taking place in business-to-business markets due to the increasing importance of the service sector to economies of most developed and developing countries. There is a growing shift from agriculture to industry and then to the service sector as the mainstay of most developing economies. In Africa, specifically in Ghana and Nigeria, the service sector is currently the largest contributor to GDP. Formerly, their agricultural sector, as it is applicable to other countries in Africa, was traditionally the biggest contributor to GDP. Today, the service sector has taken over from the agriculture sector in terms of growth and contribution to economic development. This clearly shows that the service sector in the modern economy is increasingly going through a significant revolutionary change.

Similarly, globalization has become the standard in the service industry. This is evident by a growing number of businesses that operate in more than one country and have evolved their business practices. The recorded changes in the world economy and business practices have created a new focus on service, as services dominate the modern economies of the world. The emphasis on services to be used as a competitive business advantage fulfills specific needs of the deregulated and proficient service industries; the role of new service concepts are increasing from technological advances; and the understanding that the unique characteristics of services result in unique challenges.

## The Importance of Differences Among Services

Services have become a vital part of the world economy, and over the past decade, the role of services marketing has become a prevailing feature in the service industry, particularly among developing countries. Organizations no longer regard services as an alternative to the provision of goods to society, but instead as a necessity to gain a competitive advantage in a contemporary information-rich world. Consequently, service firms are pursuing proper marketing of their services by providing quality and timely services in response to the increased service demand from customers. While it stands true that the kinds of services that are provided in the service sector are broad and varied, there is also the need to acknowledge that when these services are properly marketed, it results in unprecedented benefits that lead to development and achievement of organizational objectives. The next section discusses types of services.

### *Types of Services*

**Consumer Services**

The main purpose of consumer services is to provide services to individual consumers who demand them. Consumer services can come in the form of retail or personalized services, depending on the mode of service delivery.

**Retail and Wholesale Services**

Businesses in the retail and wholesale sector have been instrumental in the business environment in most economies. They make it possible for products, and in this context, services, to reach the final consumers. A typical example of retail and wholesale service businesses in the Ghanaian context is the "electricity vending" business (who work on behalf of the Ghana Grid Company—GRIDco) from whom consumers purchase electricity.

**Health Services**

In recent times, there have been efforts by several governments to improve the health sector. As such, most governments are increasing expenditure on the health sector. This is because there is a link between the general health of a country's workforce and productivity (Mitchell & Bates, 2011). This signifies the relevance of health services across nations. Businesses that offer health services include hospitals, clinics, health centers, laboratories, and pharmacies.

**Leisure and Hospitality Services**

These are the types of services performed for consumers' relaxation and comfort. Increasingly, people are becoming interested in leisure and taking vacations all over the world (Torkildsen, 2012). Hence, it is expected that this sector continues to witness significant growth.

**Business Services**

The main purpose of business services is to facilitate other businesses to produce adequate results. The services offered under this category are professional services, financial services, transportation services, and public services.

- *Professional Services:* Jobs in technical services, including law, accounting, architecture, engineering, design, and consulting are all part of professional services. This category also extends to support services, such as clerical, secretarial, and custodial work.
- *Financial Services:* This group is often called FIRE, an acronym for finance, insurance, and real estate. Financial services jobs are mostly found in banks and other financial institutions, as well as in insurance companies and real estate.
- *Transportation and Similar Services:* Businesses that diffuse and distribute services are grouped as transportation and information services. One half of these services are in transportation, primarily trucking. The other half is in information services, including publishing and broadcasting, as well as utilities such as water and electricity.
- *Public services:* Public services provide security and protection for citizens and businesses. These include teaching and other services related to federal and local government.

## The Importance of Marketing Healthcare Services

The benefits derived from the marketing of services are enormous, both to the service providers and receivers. Differentiation in product offerings in contemporary times is becoming clear. As a result, services are increasingly becoming the key differentiators of offerings in the minds of consumers. For example, considering two fast-food chains that serve similar products (Pizza Hut® and Domino's®), beyond just the product, the quality of service rendered by these two businesses will be used by consumers in differentiating the two brands. Therefore, services can be leveraged by marketers as a differentiation element from the competition and attract consumers.

In marketing service, relationship building is key to success. Considering that the product is intangible, most customers will make their decisions to buy depending on the extent to which they trust the seller. Hence, marketers must listen to the needs of the customer and fulfill them through the appropriate service offering and build a long-lasting relationship, which might lead to repeat sales and positive word-of-mouth.

Given today's highly competitive environment where several healthcare providers are targeting a limited pool of customers, customer retention has become more relevant than the efforts to attract new ones. Since the production and consumption of healthcare services occur simultaneously, customers become involved in the service delivery process by specifying their service requirements and by offering feedback. Thus, healthcare service providers are able to provide customized services according to customer requirements, which may lead to increased satisfaction and higher customer retention.

Service marketing is the bedrock of marketing healthcare services. Healthcare providers can benefit from using services marketing concepts and theories (e.g., service quality zone of tolerance, levels of consumer satisfaction, the branding of services, patient participation, and service recovery) in order to achieve patient satisfaction and loyalty and remain competitive in today's market economy (Corbin, Kelley, & Schwartz, 2001).

## Integrating Marketing With Other Functions in Healthcare Organization

An organization cannot successfully achieve its desired objectives when it fails to effectively coordinate and integrate the various organizational functions in its strategic planning process. The individual units of an organization such as research and development, operations, human resources, and marketing and sales, all play separate but cumulative roles that contribute toward the accomplishment of the general organizational goals of business firms. It is worth noting that what happens in each of the individual departments of an organization, in terms of failures and successes in operation, have either direct or indirect bearing on the functioning of the other units. Hence, there is a need to critically analyze the relationship that exists among these functional areas and how they can be positively integrated to achieve organizational success.

According to Rouziès et al. (2005), the response to increased competitive pressures, the shortening of product life cycles, and heightened customer demands are the reasons businesses are increasing their ability to effectively adapt and build competitive advantage by going horizontal— flattening their organizations, breaking down barriers between functions, and stimulating more teamwork between functional areas. Similarly, Kim and Lee (2010) are of the opinion that many factors such as cost reduction, speed of new product development, on-time delivery, reduction in inventory, and a better interface between/among organizational functions are some of the factors that are calling for the integration of marketing of services with other organizational functions.

It is essential for people in charge of strategy development and implementation in service firms to carefully infuse decisions regarding all the functional units of the service firm in a way that promotes information flow and coordination of activities among these departments. For instance, the service marketing department thrives on information from the research and development department. In the same way, the operations department always uses data obtained by the service marketing department for decisions regarding the volume to be produced and the type and design of particular services. This helps the organization to better provide efficient quality services to its target and potential markets. In the context of healthcare marketing, the organization must ensure that the marketing strategy cuts across every other department to make all healthcare workers carriers of this strategy. All departments must key into the broader picture of healthcare marketing, which is expected to influence all service plans and activities. Integrating marketing with other functions in the organization will change the modus operandi and influence the provision of quality healthcare service delivery. Marketing healthcare service cannot work in isolation; therefore, it must speak through all other departments within the healthcare organization, to achieve the desired goal.

## Conclusion

Customers play an important role in the co-creation process of service delivery and consumption. This has, therefore, resulted in the dire need for all service industries, particularly those in fiercely competitive markets, to develop specific organization strategies with an eye on the customer. In the healthcare sector, for example, where the majority of decisions revolve around the provision of novel and outstanding services, there is the need for strategic integration of all decisions that affect the various functional units of the healthcare organization, to achieve better returns on investment. These decisions should be taken in the light of the multiple roles the individual elements in the marketing mix concept play in the provision of excellent health services. Consequently, it is necessary for health service firms to improve the service quality of their offerings for greater differentiation in today's competitive marketplace in order to stay very competitive and profitable.

## Review Questions

1. Explain what service marketing is.
2. Discuss the evolution of the service marketing concept from 4Ps to 7Ps.
3. Discuss the difference between product and services marketing.
4. Explain how these differences pose distinctive marketing challenges.

### MINI CASE STUDY: IMPROVED SERVICES AND REBRANDING STRATEGY INCREASE REVENUES FOR SMALL MEDICAL CENTER

For decades, John Medical Center (JMC) had been a small rural hospital well known for its quality of care. Located about an hour outside a large city with three major hospitals, JMC served two demographics: the rural dwellers, most of whom were born and nurtured nearby, and urban dwellers who valued the quiet and relaxed atmosphere of the sub-urban location.

Because of its location in a charming small town environment with excellent schools and a friendly atmosphere, JMC had attracted healthcare professionals who had gained a reputation for providing exceptional primary healthcare services. However, the staff agreed that they wanted to do more and, therefore, committed to months of fundraising and grant writing aimed at expanding their capacity. In a bid to become competitive with the urban hospitals and meet the healthcare needs of its community, JMC decided to rebrand itself to become known as a hospital that would deliver excellent healthcare services using the latest technology. The first step of this rebranding effort began with adopting a new name. JMC became

John Specialist Medical Center (JSMC). Other elements of the rebranding campaign followed:

1. a logo change,
2. a website redesign,
3. a community-wide health seminar chaired by the Commissioner of Health,
4. partnership with an Indian hospital,
5. internal employee buy-in, and
6. a new tagline, "Outstanding Healthcare Delivery, Always."

The new JSMC brand attracted the attention of specialists who were trained at prominent medical centers from around the world and who decided to practice at JSMC. Patients were assured of receiving excellent healthcare delivery in a welcoming environment. Within 7 years, JSMC became an internationally known medical center that drew patients from both rural and urban communities.

The launch of John Specialist Medical Center's award-winning brand generated the largest increase in outpatient revenue in the hospital's history.

### Discussion Questions

1. Identify and describe three marketing strategies John Specialist Medical Center should adopt to achieve the goals established by the hospital administration.
2. JSMC is located in a rural community. Give two positive and two negative potential impacts that location could have on the hospital's rebranding efforts. Include ways the hospital could capitalize on the positive aspects of its location and ways that it could overcome the negative aspects.

## References

Baruch, J. J., Quinn, J. B., Penny, C., & Paquette, P. C. (1987). Technology in services. *Scientific American, 257*(6), 50–59.

Berenson, R. A., & Rich, E. C. (2010). US approaches to physician payment: the deconstruction of primary care. *Journal of General Internal Medicine, 25*(6), 613–618.

Berry, L. L., & Parasuraman, A. (2004). *Marketing services: Competing through quality.* New York, NY: Simon and Schuster.

Booms, B. H., & Bitner, M. J. (1981). Marketing strategies and organization structures for service firms. *Marketing of Services, 25*(3), 47–52.

Corbin, C. L., Kelley, S. W., & Schwartz, R. W. (2001). Concepts in service marketing for healthcare professionals. *The American Journal of Surgery, 181*(1), 1–7.

Dominici, G. (2009). From marketing mix to e-marketing mix: A literature overview and classification. *International Journal of Business and Management, 4*(9), 17–24.

Gronroos, C. (1994). From marketing mix to relationship marketing: Towards a paradigm shift in marketing. *Asia-Australia Marketing Journal, 2*(1), 9–29.

Irons, K. (1997). *The world of superservice: Creating profit through a passion for customer service.* Reading, MA: Addison-Wesley.

Kent, R. A. (1986). Faith in four Ps: An alternative. *Journal of Marketing Management, 2*(2), 145–154.

Kotler, P. (2000). Marketing management: The millennium edition. *Marketing Management, 23*(6), 188–193.

Kotler, P. (2002). *Marketing places.* New York, NY: Simon and Schuster.

Lovelock, C. H., Patterson, P. G., & Walker, R. H. (1998*). Marketing services: Australia-New Zealand.* Sydney, Australia: Prentice-Hall.

Mitchell, V. W., & Greatorex, M. (1993). Risk perception and reduction in the purchase of consumer services. *Service Industries Journal, 13*(4), 179–200.

Mitchell, R. J., & Bates, P. (2011). Measuring health-related productivity loss. *Population Health Management, 14*(2), 93–98.

Rouziès, D., Anderson, E., Kohli, A. K., Michaels, R. E., Weitz, B. A., & Zoltners, A. A. (2005). Sales and marketing integration: A proposed framework. *Journal of Personal Selling & Sales Management, 25*(2), 113–122.

Smith, K. T. (2017). Hospital marketing and communications via social media. *Services Marketing Quarterly, 38*(3), 187–201.

Soriya, S., & Dhaigude, A. S. (2016). Corporate online reporting and their determinants in Indian services sector. In *Handbook of research on promotional strategies and consumer influence in the service sector* (pp. 355–370). Hershey, PA: IGI Global.

Strydom, J. (Ed.). (2005). *Introduction to marketing.* Cape Town, South Africa: Juta and Company.

Torkildsen, G. (2012). *Leisure and recreation management.* New York, NY: Routledge.

Van Waterschoot, W., & Van den Bulte, C. (1992). The 4P classification of the marketing mix revisited. *The Journal of Marketing, 56*(4), 83–93.

Vargo, S. L., & Lusch, R. F. (2008). From goods to service(s): Divergences and convergences of logics. *Industrial marketing management, 37*(3), 254–259.

Zeithaml, V., A., & Bitner, M. J. (2000), Services marketing: Integrating customer focus across the firm (2nd ed.). Boston, MA: Irwin/McGraw-Hill.

# 3

## *The Evolving Societal and Healthcare Context*

### Chapter Outline

- Introduction
- The Evolution of Healthcare
- The Cultural Revolution and Healthcare
- The Changing Societal Context
- The Country Context
- The Emergence of Healthcare as an Institution
- Marketing Concepts for Healthcare Organizations
- Components of the Healthcare Marketing Mix
- Conclusion
- Review Questions
- Mini Case Study With Discussion Questions
- References

*Marketing in Healthcare-Related Industries*, pages 45–75
Copyright © 2020 by Information Age Publishing
All rights of reproduction in any form reserved.

## Chapter Outcome

By the end of this chapter, the reader will be able to

- explain the evolution of healthcare,
- discuss the emergence of healthcare as an institution,
- discuss how the changing societal setup affects healthcare marketing,
- discuss the different alliances in marketing healthcare, and
- describe the components of healthcare marketing.

## Introduction

The concept of healthcare has been a necessity for mankind since its inception in the 20th century and has gone through changes for many decades. All over the world, healthcare has been administered in various ways based on the perceptions and beliefs of people in different demographic areas. Various developments, mostly in the United States, set the foundation for the advent of healthcare amongst societies (Thomas, 2004). The circumstances in which people go through the human life cycle, that is, birth, growth, work, and aging can be termed as the social factors of health. The sharing of money, power, and resources worldwide molds these conditions across nations. There is, therefore, discrimination and unnecessary differences in health status amongst countries (Basics for Health, 2018). Also, the type of healthcare received by various groups of people can be dependent on the income, types of occupation, and educational levels in society. Those living in improved conditions receive better healthcare than those in poverty-stricken societies. Since the 19th century, there have been disparities in healthcare between the rich and poor (Te Ara Encyclopedia of New Zealand, 2018).

As the world evolves, many things need to be reconsidered and reexamined as a result of dynamism and the growing demands of human society. Many of these things include and point to value as the benchmark with human beings constituting the jury. It is now essential for organizations and institutions to harness their internal abilities in the face of external forces by aligning their interest (usually in the form of profits) to the changing needs of their customers, hence, providing better products and services. One issue worthy of note here is the subject of healthcare. This is a fundamental service which must perpetually improve, be invested in, and must be allocated appropriately in a way that benefits the various markets it serves and the healthcare organization as a whole. The primary focus of the healthcare organization is the value it offers which will be highlighted in two ways: disease prevention and health promotion.

## The Evolution of Healthcare

Healthcare began with individual private hospitals offering services on a prepaid basis and has evolved into the health insurance systems found in many countries. Amidst these changes are also evolving factors pertaining to the societies that receive the services. The social classes of people from the lower to the upper classes have over the years received healthcare in different ways or at different levels; and the fact remains that some are better than others, dependent on the lifestyle changes. The healthcare field is transforming daily with emerging trends in utilization patterns; the science of medicine; technology; increased information; payment models and policy, competition, partners and collaborators; engagement and behavior change; and the holistic view of the population's health. For example, patient care continues to move from inpatient to outpatient settings due to cost savings and the availability of new medical technologies. This has set a center stage for marketing in healthcare. Gradually, healthcare is centered more on creating policies to improve the quality delivered to the populace as opposed to quality improvement in the earlier periods that were derived from a series of incidents and developments that had no association whatsoever (Sheingold & Hahn, 2014).

In the effort to deliver the best services to create health value and equity for patients, the sector has grown and made better expansions in most of its practices, especially in the United States. These include teaching methods, technology usage, marketing strategies, and standard practices of health providers or practitioners, to mention a few. Patients alongside have also evolved from being unable to afford good healthcare services to accessing current health insurance policies run by many governments.

## The Cultural Revolution and Healthcare

Bowden and Smits (2012) assert that culture is the accumulated results of a defined group's experience-based learning, communicated to new members to help them cope with external challenges and operate cohesively as a group. The common beliefs and values practiced by a group of people become part of them over time. Culture also becomes difficult to change and more influential when it is reinforced by various actions. There are different levels of cultures consisting of geographic, organizational, and occupational cultures. Healthcare institutions operate mostly in organizational and occupational cultures all over the world.

Organizational culture works as a domain in the leadership of organizations and has an impact on important aspects such as performance and change management. Therefore, culture can be said to be the "organization's immune system." It protects the organization from the entry of disturbing actions while helping in regulating operations by identifying changes that may appear to be attacks to the organization.

Occupational culture sees the employment of a variety of occupational groups to successfully discharge the processes that create value. Persons receiving healthcare services deal with multiple professionals, each with its own educational requirements; technical language; treatment modalities and regimes; and standards of practice, ethical codes, and traditions that cumulatively evolve into a professional culture. There are types of culture that healthcare institutions dwell on as part of their identity. These are the culture of perfection, silence, and autonomy, and they are significant when it comes to shame and medical error.

Scripts and logic are used to measure the standard performance of physicians as a culture of perfection in their training stages. Meanwhile, that of silence dictates how a physician should react to a medical error, and the culture of autonomy teaches physicians how to behave with their patients and coworkers (Jarvis, 2016).

Using shared knowledge, culture can thrive at various degrees of organized actions. When success is recorded in practicing a behavior, it is imparted into fresh members by interactive measures. This teaches the employee how to understand, ponder, be aware, and conduct himself/herself in a society. New directions have set into the healthcare culture all over the world, thereby, causing decisive and exemplary changes. When new trends gain a strong standing and start challenging the old culture, the latter will become weak. These changes may take a long time to be implemented, but the discretion of people will begin to have an adverse effect on the behavior and perceptions consistently. Some people are of the opinion that healthcare will not go through much changes scientifically, technologically, service wise or systems wise; business models will, however, become more advanced and regulatory oversight will remain a persisting bug in the health industry. They rather believe the institution needs a new culture of change that befits the intricate and ever-changing properties it possesses. This type of culture will always be in expectation of change and will be easily managed to merge efficiently with other institutions as well (Bowden & Smits, 2012).

Based on visits from family physicians in the early days, some cultural expectations were established which evolved into the existing healthcare system. These consisted of trust, privacy, personalized care, and professionalism. Likewise, discoveries made in the science and technology fields that save, extend, and improve the lives of patients have basically changed the underbuilding and administration of healthcare (Bowden & Smits, 2012). Emphasis has been placed on the original model of modern Western medicine, which was supported by new values coming out of World War II in the United States and which helped develop the healthcare system. There was at that time an encounter of growth in terms of economic profitability, educational improvements, and scientific and technological milestones clocked in the United States afterward. Before the era of World War II, health was perceived as not being a value but just a notion of well-being. This perception has changed in the 21st century, where health is now viewed as a value that is promoting healthcare institutions (Thomas, 2004). All these types of culture play important roles in the evolution of healthcare.

## The Changing Societal Context

The 20th century generated a reliance on various types of formal institutions, thereby, creating a favorable environment for the emergence of a strong healthcare system. There were several demographic changes in various aspects of societies pertaining to healthcare systems by the end of the 20th century. Areas that saw a change in trends were the age structure, household and family structure, and consumer attitudes. The healthcare sector, therefore, faced complex challenges arising from advances in medical treatment, heightened needs and demands from patients, and decreasing resources to fund healthcare (Crepaldi, De Rosa, & Pesce, 2012). Trends that have evolved over the years include:

### Demographic Trends

Demographic trends (e.g., age, gender, ethnicity, education) affect healthcare demand and cost. Thus, healthcare organizations need to be responsive to these changes. For example, the U.S. population is aging, which has created demand for specialized services such as home healthcare, palliative care, and hospice care. Thus, healthcare providers in the United States are already adapting and responding to changing demographics. Research has shown that education has a significant role to play in healthcare utilization; educated consumers are more likely to use healthcare services. The minority racial and ethnic groups, especially of Hispanic origin, are growing rapidly in the United States, and this demographic shift may challenge healthcare delivery systems. Providers unaccustomed to caring for diverse groups of patients who might have distinct needs must adapt to such demographic changes. To address this trend, cultural competency training for healthcare professionals and organizations has been recognized as a key strategy to reduce racial and ethnic disparities in access to and quality of healthcare and patient outcomes (Dell'Aversana & Bruno, 2017). Cultural competency is the ability of systems to provide care to patients with diverse values, beliefs, and behaviors, and this includes tailoring delivery to meet patients' social, cultural, and linguistic needs (Betancourt, Green, & Carrillo, 2002). The demographic trends are key to the understanding of the population dynamics. These alterations of the population in the 20th century needed to be tackled by the healthcare system. In documented history, severe conditions added up to become major health threats and became the major causes of death. This slowly changed during the second part of the 20th century. The new demographic trends led to a shift away from acute conditions and toward chronic conditions as the predominant form of health problems. Later in that century, the population saw an improvement in the living conditions, nutrition, and standards of living, while there was a significant enhancement in medical science that reduced or eliminated the burden of disease from acute conditions (Thomas, 2004).

### Age Structure

Age is presumably the most important indicator of demand for health services, and this is known because the trend for the demand for health services is documented. The prevalence of chronic diseases, physical disabilities, mental illnesses, and other co-morbidities are expected to grow with an aging population (Boutayeb & Boutayeb, 2005). Healthcare expenses rise with age because an aging population is the major utilizer of healthcare products and services. An aging population needs long-term care, which promote patients' physical, mental, social, and spiritual well-being and maximizes their quality of life. For example, growth in population among those within age 55 and above, is on the rise in the United States, and this will have a major implication on the U.S. healthcare system. The trend has already created an imbalance in the demand and supply of hospital services and healthcare professionals. A constant shortage of younger cohorts, that is, mostly the working class (between 25 and 40) continued until the baby boom cohorts reached this age. This group of individuals was brought up in riches and comfort, and so they were used to getting things, including healthcare. The baby boomers are today's aging population. The healthcare system was tremendously affected when they had to contend with the onset of chronic diseases and natural deterioration. The growth of this aging group was during the marketing era, and so they are more comfortable with marketing healthcare than generations that preceded them.

## *Household and Family Structure*

Family systems have seen major changes in rates of new marriages, divorce rates, and procreation rates. Changes in line with marital status have had huge impacts on household structures. Just like marital status, a change in household structure has repercussions on both health behavior and health status. For example, children in step relationships, children of single mothers, or children of grandparent-only families are less likely to have a physician visit, and they have poorer health than children living with two biological parents (Bramlett & Blumberg, 2007). The constant modification of the household system has, thus, seen an appreciable diversification in the healthcare delivery system. This has led to the provision of employer-sponsored insurance coverage in many companies for their employees alongside the national health insurance policies put in place by various governments. In total, new marketing approaches have been developed, targeting the family as standards using customary marketing tactics.

## *Consumer Attitudes*

Patients' attitudes toward health, healthcare services, and healthcare providers appear to be changing significantly. In the 21st century, consumers are seen to measure healthcare by approaching it from both their own behavior and the institution's perspective. Some go through a scientific approach to decide where to receive medical care or prevention, while others measure healthcare and make judgments based on demographic attributes, ranks, and perception of the institutions (Gould, 2018). Consumers are currently helped to make informed choices concerning their personal healthcare by a trend known as the consumer reports. These reports have helped improve the attitudes of healthcare professionals and their services. It is suggested that consumer behavior has a significant role to play in healthcare and these consumer reports give real strategies to improve the worth of patient care (Longo, Land, & Wayne Schramm, 1997).

## The Country Context

Healthcare provision is important, irrespective of the location; however, in the context of healthcare management, it is essential to understand the country context and how it shapes the marketing and management strategy, especially with regards to government provision and healthcare insurance.

### Countries With Insurance Funded Healthcare

The United States will be a good example of this. There are numerous insurance companies and managed care organizations that market various types of insurance plans targeted to different market segments with minimum government interference or regulation. Marketing can play a key role in the health insurance market by informing consumers about the availability of different insurance plans, particularly where hospitals are run as commercial ventures, as there is a well-structured health insurance scheme that can support the industry. Since the access to healthcare services is particularly based on insurance coverage, patients use the hospital they can afford, depending on their insurance coverage. This allows the hospital to position themselves to target unique demographics; they advertise and market themselves because they want to target premium customers. The negative implication of this system cannot be overlooked. Some individuals who do not have the insurance or the right insurance coverage may end up not receiving care because they cannot afford to pay the private hospital bills.

### Countries With Government Funded Healthcare

The United Kingdom will be an example of this case. The United Kingdom's public universal health system, the National Health Services (NHS), emphasizes the free point of access and equal access in which people are guaranteed that they will receive needed healthcare and consequently, they would not often need private health insurance. This also influences the advertising strategies of these organizations. They do not usually advertise to treat but to prevent, they do more of social marketing to create public awareness and reduce the stress on the NHS. They advertise and advise people to stop smoking, to stop driving drunk rather than going to accident and emergency wards, and also to take their flu shot. However, the negative effect of this system cannot be ignored—it causes a huge financial strain on the government, as people are living longer and with different medical conditions, it takes a toll on the budget. This is inadvertently leading to a growing market for private healthcare. For those who want healthcare that is not being covered by the NHS or cannot afford to wait for the long referral, they use their private health insurance or pay privately for the services consumed. This triggers private healthcare providers to utilize the advertising services to create awareness of available medical services to meet the growing and unique needs. These needs could range from emergency, general, and special procedures such as cosmetics surgeries, in vitro fertilization (IVF), and nursing care for the elderly, among others.

### *Countries With Privately Funded Healthcare*

Customers often pay for their own healthcare under a National Health Insurance Scheme (NHIS). NHIS is a tax-supported mechanism through which the government guarantees a basic package of health services to all citizens. The scheme is sometimes not well funded in some countries where it is operational. An example is the NHIS of Nigeria, which was founded in 1999, and that of Ghana, founded in 2003. The healthcare sector, in this case, is not well funded by the government and as a result, customers rely greatly on private organizations to provide the needed healthcare. This highlights the marketing challenges for healthcare providers in Africa. With the understanding of the market, the need for healthcare provision, and the financial capabilities of their customer base, how can they effectively target their customers and still be commercially viable? Since the government may not be making many contributions through the insurance scheme, the expenses fall on the customers and their family members who may need to raise money for their healthcare bills. This issue is more evident in developing countries.

## The Emergence of Healthcare as an Institution

The development of hospitals symbolized the institutionalization of healthcare and became the central core around which the delivery of medical services was organized (Shi & Singh, 2017; Torrens, 1993). Healthcare has advanced into scientifically structured processes with more complicated technology, and hence, pays more attention to caregiving processes (Bowden & Smits, 2012). Within a span of 20 years, conveyance and funding in caregiving have changed massively. There has also been a rise in therapeutic fields, alongside a group of pharmaceuticals. Care delivery moved basically from inpatient locations to a stylish environment that serves as an outpatient setting. The way of supporting care has also been changed, as accomplished care has become a leading piece of the health institution (Thomas, 2004).

Healthcare in the 21st century has experienced a move in the operating system of service-based processes to a population-based process. The responsibility of a healthcare professional now lies with taking care of the population in their geographical territory as opposed to the earlier practice where they provided services to people who demanded their help. The eventful move has brought about more innovations to help achieve the new objectives of the healthcare institutions. In recent years, decisions have been made concerning the type of healthcare service delivered to the different types of customers or consumers. Managers currently have targets to be met to grow their organizations' capacity for customers, including all people in the institution's locality. Health workers are, therefore, entreated to brainstorm and help management introduce ways to liaise with other organizations in their territory (Breton, Lamothe, & Denis, 2014).

Education is very crucial to the success of innovations in an institution. Due to this phenomenon, managers are required to have a higher level of education to be able to handle issues pertaining to the development of their institutions. Healthcare amenities assume mastery of skills acquired in higher education such as a master's degree in healthcare administration and managerial skills that are almost inborn for leaders. A leader's ability to assimilate with his subordinates and to realize their goals and objectives is very important, hence, this new operational trend's evolvement (Utica College, 2018). The old system of healthcare saw physicians dictating procedures and pay structures. This has been transformed with the objective of giving less costly care as well as better quality to developing a whole system of services in clinical and organizational platforms. These changes have had an adverse effect on organizational populations and structural processes (Light, 2002).

The healthcare system is currently difficult compared to previous years. Recorded changes show a move from the focus of professionals viewing their responsibilities as mere obligations, dependent on the wants of patients to a managed care practice. For example, healthcare in the United States has been transformed within a space of a couple of generations and yet is still improving. To consider the newness of operations of a healthcare institution, managers must look at the factors causing change, the difference in healthcare between past and present, the significance of the changes, what trends an organization should adopt, and the results to be incurred in the future. These questions are very necessary as humans continue to age, incurring more costs in the bid to receive better healthcare, while treatment prices shoot up; hence, a few people need to receive healthcare support (Thomas, 2004).

General practitioners now liaise with other health workers to form the primary health organization in the 21st century. In the 1940s, patients had to settle their bills for health services delivered, and the deprived ones received free treatments that were partly funded at public hospitals. This meant that the general practitioners fixed their own fees, while some societies received subsidized bills because they were regulars at the health institutions. Unlike this era, the new dawn has brought the NHIS, run by governments of many countries (Te Ara Encyclopedia of New Zealand, 2018).

Pertaining to regulations in healthcare, there has been a drastic change from the 19th century to date. Many countries operated systems where healthcare providers controlled their entry and exit procedures, but that is not the case today. Healthcare authorities now make use of improved answerability as a new trend to regulate these professionals in the 21st century. Therefore, there has been an increase in the number of regulatory bodies and strategies to complement and manage prevailing professional self-regulation systems. The various changes have been realized because of the weakened trust patients have built for the former self-regulated system, that was characterized by prominent medical scandals (Beaupert et al., 2014).

Patient privacy has gained attention and recognition recently due to breaches and violations of different forms. This has enlightened patients more on their privacy rights when it comes to healthcare. Customers currently deem it very important to refer to privacy and security guidelines before receiving services from a healthcare institution. Patients view privacy protection as a deciding factor in healthcare selection alongside other determinants such as cost, the admissions processes, and quality of service received in hospitals. This has put management on top of their game to deliver quality service to their customers in terms of privacy policies (Utica College, 2018).

The ideas and thoughts of patients were largely considered unimportant before the 1980s, when healthcare moved to the adoption of marketing strategies. Subsequently, it became very necessary for healthcare providers and practitioners to know patients' preferences in their services. Various researches were carried out to find ways to satisfy patients, and medical surveys were conducted frequently. In implementing findings and improving on limitations from these research works, healthcare professionals and their processes received grades on report cards to assess their outputs. Marketers were employed to help the institutions to know what their patients needed and wanted, as well as the processes of maintaining the degrees of customer fulfillment they had attained (Sheingold & Hahn, 2014).

Data collection is a necessary process in the healthcare field. Over the years, health providers have evolved the various ways of accumulating data from patients. In recent times, new processes have been initiated to help the easy collection and manipulation of data, that is, information about patients. This was created to improve the impact of customer experience in the institutions and also to gain loyalty from customers. The introduction of automated systems helps clinicians to go through large numbers of data in real-time, and also, it gives the best patient experiences. These systems are of different types. They keep records of post-visit feedback surveys and peak and off-peak service delivery days, so managers can staff their offices adequately. The new forms of data can, for example, predict periods when patients will get sick to put in preventive measures. It can also be done on a personalized level (Morgan, 2018).

Social media is a global-growing platform used by current healthcare practitioners to get closer to their present and prospective patients. Healthcare facilities have formed alliances to introduce serviceable platforms such as infographics, videos, and slideshows for customers and the general public to help them in their health issues. In addition to this, hospitals distribute research information, news, and events updates on these social media platforms with patients and employees. There is also an increase in the number of people surfing the web to link with other users who share the same interest in healthcare, while searching for friends who will help and support in their circumstances (Utica College, 2018).

With the issue of efficiency, managers have started employing measures to curb the incidences of readmissions in their institutions. Many facilities have started using healthcare management logics to curtail readmissions, and the practice is increasing with speed in most institutions. The providers or practitioners have realized the need for a relationship between the number of people who visit healthcare institutions daily and the chances of readmissions, and so, are paying attention to those factors that can be avoided. By decreasing the chances of readmissions, costs and patient waiting times are lessened, and healthcare professionals become less busy so they can take on more shifts with patients. (Utica College, 2018).

Within 20 to 30 years, improvements achieved in the healthcare industry have seen the patient as the center, holding all activities concerning the marketing of healthcare together. It is postulated that the word *patient* meant more by the 20th century, and hence, today it is used less. It has since been replaced with a few other words, such as client, customer, consumer, or enrollee. Demands from these customers have brought additional attention from healthcare professionals and have developed partnerships in the management of healthcare institutions. This has caused a positive shift in healthcare marketing to other industries.

Healthcare systems operate differently in various societies. Institutions consist of categories of systems, working together to achieve societal goals. In trying to see to the every day recurring personal needs of people in a society, these institutions gradually evolve to become stable. The history that revolves around the culture of a society, its surroundings, links between societies, and its demographic features, help in building an institution (Thomas, 2004). Mohrman and Shani (2014) add that the extent to which change can bring sustainability to a healthcare system is minimal because new methods evolve daily. In recent years, there has been much effort by several bodies to see the transformation of the healthcare institution from professional dominance to giving integrated care (Light, 2002).

Being effective and efficient is a big challenge to workers in the public health system worldwide (Mesabbah & Arisha, 2016). Many organizations dealing in healthcare try to bridge the gap between services rendered and available resources, while making an effort to improve on the quality they deliver to patients in general. In trying to introduce new systems into existing complex ones, such as healthcare, one can sometimes face oppositions from varied levels. Rules are formed to serve as guides for people who find themselves to be part of the healthcare institutions. For example, policies have been placed to deliver long life to patients. If these guidelines are not followed, people risk losing their lives to sicknesses. These principles are often termed as "doctor's orders."

During the 1900s, doctors were feared by patients with the notion that hospitals caused the death of sick persons who reported to the facilities. Seeking medical attention was generally undesirable except in times of serious need, but this trend began changing in the 21st century. There has been an increase in the number of doctors in most nations due to the realization of the need for these professionals in healthcare institutions. This has made them a very important part of society in most countries (Thomas, 2004). In enforcing stable institutions in the healthcare industry, the ideology of shame as a corrective mechanism has been adopted. This works by reinforcing norms that pertain to the identities of physicians. The mechanism is a part of organizational culture and works such that, a medical error leaves a physician's reputation tarnished and induces a feeling of personal failure. The physicians are taught this type of working culture during their socialization into the medical profession (Jarvis, 2016).

Healthcare has traditionally been delivered solely on considering how cost-efficient it is rather than focusing on the value a patient derives from each service received. Patient value must be recognized as the most important driver to be considered in improving healthcare for societies and even for individuals. Management of the entire care process must see an improvement while measuring the value of every outcome from the micro to macro levels in the bid to give quality care. This means that healthcare as an institution must be efficient in using value creation as a strategy to achieve rolling out the best care services in every society (Gambarov, Sarno, Hysa, Calabrese, & Bilotta, 2017). In practicing industrialization and urbanization, healthcare has been developed and has become one of the institutions that give the best value to patients dependent on formal solutions. This institution has also received many essential resources from other industries, thereby, making it very important in political circles.

The emerging issues in health, beauty, and fitness have witnessed significant changes in the last decade, giving rise to a boom in advertisements and paid programming in the media circles. While health products and services are taking over advertising through television ads, health institutions are also dominating through health issues being featured on paid programs such as fitness training and devoted programs aired on television (Thomas, 2004). Recently, information on healthcare has also been made easily accessible on the Internet as part of evolvement in the media arena. Websites are being developed every day to provide information to consumers concerning varied/various topics in healthcare.

In moving forward, organizations are consciously making an effort to broaden their knowledge and utilize the measurement information in their decision-making processes. In order to achieve their objectives of giving the best healthcare services to their clients, Porter et al. (2016) in Nordin, Kork, and Koskela (2017) admonished healthcare institutions to implement technological structures to help solve problems in their decision-making processes too. In trying to give quality to attain improvement in services rendered, patient value is seen to be the most essential part of the healthcare processes. Healthcare practitioners can focus on giving value to patients during the care process on interventions promoting multi-professional care. Porter (2010) believes that the benefits derived from interventions usually depend on the effectiveness and efficiency of previous interventions carried out for patient outcomes. The delivery of healthcare in recent years has seen the empowerment of patients and support of clinical decision-making to be the sources of improvement in quality.

With the introduction of new health information technologies to bring a change in modern healthcare services, patient outcomes can be measured and improved. This will allow staff of various healthcare institutions to use, collect, and aggregate data to keep in check and measure their performances and know how to maintain their achievements (Black, 2013). The strategies used can be disease-oriented (how specific treatments are estimated) or generic (how the quality of a patient's life is determined).

Organizations are now paying more attention to patient engagement than they do with the professionals in achieving their aims and objectives during recent years (Nordin et al., 2017). Incentives are given to health practitioners to keep them on their toes in delivering excellent health services for the institutions to have a competitive edge over their rivals. It is possible for healthcare providers to create incentives as part of their human resource strategies, but there is very little evidence of how these incentives help the outcomes of services rendered, pertaining to the improvement in the business being run and the health values provided for consumers. In trying to shift the institutions to a value-based system, learning has become expedient throughout the organizational practice. This is done by improving effectiveness throughout the caregiving cycle instead of through cost reduction (Nordin et al., 2017).

Currently, most hospitals are employing the concept of *benchmarking* to deliver the best services to patients. In trying to maintain an excellent management output in healthcare institutions, benchmarking is employed as a tool for improvement. This enables them to attain a level of quality output while they care, satisfy, or delight their patients. When expectations are met or exceeded, management is able to contain and reduce costs in their processes, too (von Eiff, 2015). Some of these practices are:

- self-measurement of periodic key performance indicators,
- measurement of key performance indicators in comparison with competitors,
- identification of best practices,
- equalizing or exceeding accepted best practice in the health sector, and
- focusing on uncomplicated and efficient processes to carry out solutions to problems.

Additionally, loyalty programs help healthcare institutions to grow their customer loyalty and equity in the society. Marketers use great concepts such as loyalty cards, frequent guest programs, and bonus programs as ways of rolling out loyalty schemes to attract and maintain patients, while increasing the acuity in both micro and macro levels. This can be done by means of actively working hand in hand to raise value (Gambarov et al., 2017).

## Marketing Concepts for Healthcare Organizations

In order to gain a deep understanding of the adoption of marketing concepts by healthcare organizations, it is imperative to examine the network in which the healthcare system operates. It includes not only their customers, but also third parties (insurers), other healthcare providers (colleagues/competitors/referrers), authorities (local, regional, national), and stakeholders, all of which drive a need and expect value. The right balance between the interrelationship within the network and the implication for adopting the marketing concepts will be analyzed in this section. The caveat here is that the network model is based on the Dutch healthcare system, which also represents many healthcare systems under regulated competitions (Boonekamp, 1994).

## The Alliance With Internal and External Customers

In terms of profit, there is an alliance of exchange that exists between providers and consumers. The former, offering the service and the latter using it and paying for it later. Translating the same concept into the healthcare sector is not feasible because there is no direct relationship between the provider and the consumer. A clear distinction can, therefore, be made that the consumer is the individual who actually receives the service, and the customer is the organization who pays for the service (Hayden, 1993). Furthermore, the value any consumer expects from a healthcare organization can be described with respect to the reduction of uncertainty, pain, injury, restoring the person to normal form, vaccination, immunization, and information aimed at preventive healthcare service. In order to develop a lasting relationship with consumers, healthcare organizations need to meet the requirements of consumers to develop trust in the organization, which can lead to customer loyalty (Boonekamp, 1994). The provision of healthcare service can be seen in two dimensions: tangible, that is, the result of the service and intangible, that is, the delivery of the service (e.g., physical evidence, queueing system, etc.). Due to the complex nature of the former, consumers usually base their opinions of quality on the physical component of the service.

The implication for adopting the marketing concept is that the expectations of the consumers and the perception they have of the value the healthcare system renders significantly affect the marketing strategy of the healthcare system. It is not enough to concentrate only on the intangible dimension of the service, but great efforts also must be put in the tangible nature as it is based on this that consumers make their judgments.

In the health sector, the primary customer is the patient. There is also, however, the internal customer. Internal customers generally are employees of a given business/organization. In this case, the internal customers of the healthcare organization are medical doctors, physician assistants, nurses, ward assistants, lab technicians, and cleaners, amongst others. It is essential that for the kind of services these internal customers offer, they are adequately equipped and motivated. Unlike other sectors where errors would only likely lead to reduced profits, in the healthcare organization, a very simple error or mismanagement of an issue can result in the loss of many lives. Thus, people who work for healthcare organizations must always be ready to offer premium quality care to the external customer—the patient. To be able to do this, they must be sufficiently resourced. State-of-the-art diagnostic and surgical equipment, friendly work climate, and commensurate remuneration are among the resources needed by these professionals to function optimally. When these are available, it becomes effortless for these professionals to offer the external customer optimal quality healthcare.

An organization that is successful at selling itself to its internal customers is about 80% successful with the external customer also. Businesses suffer losses when they fail to satisfy the needs of their internal customers, who serve the external customers. We direct our attention now to the external customer—the patient. This customer group is made up of individuals who are seeking either preventive or curative care. Preventive care is seeking medical advice/information that aids in the prevention of future ailments/conditions. Curative care, on the other hand, is seeking medical information/care/advice/procedure, in order to restore one's failed health state to normal.

Whether preventive or curative, these are people who go to hospitals, clinics, pharmacies, chemist stores, or even virtual spaces (via e-health materials) where they can acquire health information. Being unwell is hard and uncomfortable enough; what these customers need, therefore, are places where they can receive gentle and quality care. They do not need screaming nurses, ill-trained nurses, or a specialist who might misdiagnose their conditions. What they need is an understanding medical officer with whom they can trust and communicate.

Apart from these internal and external customers, there are also persons/institutions who relate closely with these healthcare organizations. We cannot call them customers; they are more in a partnership relationship with the health sector rather than a "producer–customer" relationship, as opposed to the earlier category of customers (even though patients are also partners). Partnership in this context, however, seeks to say that these people collaborate with the healthcare organization to satisfy the needs of their customers. They provide services that complement the product offerings of the health sector.

Paramount among this group of people is health insurance providers. This is largely a group of partners/customers who conceptualize, develop, and implement health payment solutions/plans which enable/aid affordability of medical solutions. Whether managed by the state or private institutions/individuals, insurance schemes make the cost of accessing healthcare lower than it would have been in the absence of the health insurance scheme. In Ghana, just like other places in the world, the state operates a scheme (NHIS), made available to all its citizenry to alleviate the burden of medical care. This health scheme has had its own share of issues in terms of effective administration at many levels, but it continues to help save precious lives at many points. Apart from the state, there are private insurance providers who tailor their service packages to the medical needs of employees of corporate institutions. In the area of administration, these private schemes work better than the state-managed kind.

In the health sector, it often becomes challenging to separate the service from the physical product offering. In fact, the service is critical to the effective and efficient delivery of the physical product. Customer service is key in the health sector. In general, being customer-oriented entails actions that appeal and keep consumers that go beyond transactions, but also develop a relationship with them (Frambach, Wels-Lips, & Gündlack, 1997).

The smiling nurse administering an injection makes a rather painful procedure/process less painful and in some cases, even pleasant. The friendliness of a medical officer makes one's medical pains and worries more bearable than they otherwise would be. These actions increasingly position the healthcare organization as the place to find solace. Health is a priority service. Many customers (patients) would go to a healthcare center to access medical care, but at the same time, when customers perceive poor quality, they are discouraged from utilizing the service (Andaleeb, 2001).

Health is key; the customer accessing any form of service in the health sector is doing so to regain lost health or prevent future ailments. It is a matter of life and death, and so it cannot be business as usual. The abysmal services enveloping the other sectors cannot continue to invade the health sector. In the end, the bigger question is, would you want to be responsible for a catastrophic outcome in your healthcare service delivery because you overlooked a basic marketing principle?

---

### The Alliance With Insurers

Insurers can be regarded as customers of a healthcare system. Therefore, relationship with them deserve the attention of healthcare organizations.

Health providers and insurers meet annually for budgetary negotiations, and the nature of their relationship is purely an administrative one. The obliged contracting system is now at its tail end, hence, providers and insurers strive for compacts. Consumers also, in tandem, possess the liberty to choose any insurer based on the most preferred policy.

Also, for insurance brokers to be competitive, they must be selective in the healthcare services they purchase so they can offer optimal policy options to consumers. The administrative nature of the third-party alliance will now take the form of a provider-purchaser relation; where negotiations will not hinge only on cost alone, but transcend to nature, place, price, and the service delivery quality (Boonekamp, 1994). This means that healthcare organizations will face the predicament of choosing between being market-driven or receptive to insurers. The implication for the adoption of the marketing concept stipulates that they should be customer-oriented to foster loyal relationships with their customers.

### Alliance With Other Healthcare Providers

Interorganizational alliances between healthcare organizations or providers is very widespread. In generic terms, there are three occurrences that can be used to explain the above. First, is the technology of the service itself. This means that, in the face of any situation where one provider is unable to attend or provide the required services of a customer, the individual is then referred to another provider or organization to provide the needed service. This will require some form of coordination and processing of the required information to prevent the customer in question from being overlooked among the referring set of healthcare organizations.

The second reason is external pressure. This is true because, for healthcare organizations to obtain resources, they usually depend on government and third parties for support, who in turn demand coordination among healthcare organizations by threats in terms of financial sanctions. The goal here is to achieve efficiency. The third reason is that relationships that exist between healthcare organizations are cooperative in nature. This can also be explained by the interorganizational culture ideology which stipulates some behavioral patterns concerning the ideal behavior with one at the far end of "competitive mode" and the other end of the "cooperative mode." Healthcare organizations, in this case, tend to portray that they are more unselfish. Hardworking professionals should always put the interest and affairs of others first. The caveat here is, despite the cooperative nature of healthcare organizations, without doubt, competition in one way or the other exists, even as they focus on customer satisfaction. This is true when the geographic services tend to overlap; hence competition may arise. An example is the differences in the quality of professionals at the various health centers within the location. The implication here for the adoption of marketing concepts by healthcare providers, is that they must be able to identify their unique value proposition (Boonekamp, 1994). This means that they should be able to work on their distinct competencies that differentiate them from the other providers, and also map them to the interest and needs of their customers. Also, a clear balance between healthcare organizations being autonomous and being interdependent should be properly ascertained.

### *Alliance With Authorities*

An important player within the network model is the government whose operations and activities transcend the different levels within the society. Healthcare in many countries is seen as so imperative for the society, that the government assumes full responsibility for assuring that this service is provided at the most basic level possible. Governments perpetually operate in the healthcare system in such countries. Even in the countries where private health insurance dominates the healthcare landscape, the government can play an important role in regulating and financing healthcare for certain uninsured and disadvantaged populations. Governments pass healthcare reforms to lower the cost and expand health insurance coverage to the uninsured population. Despite the many reforms, many countries have government-dominated healthcare systems, a typical example being the erstwhile Affordable Care Act in the United States. The government continues to play an important role within the network model by impacting the operations of the healthcare organization. These include deregulation, dominating the essence of competition, and so on. Now that it has been established that government is a significant player, healthcare organizations will have to push hard on the connections they have with government representatives, especially through persuasion. On the other hand, the implications for marketing is that, healthcare providers must also exhibit their contributions to the health sector especially on their value propositions and distinct competencies. This can be done through technology and through health professions in situations where there is strong competition for the allocation of scarce resources within the sector.

## Components of the Healthcare Marketing Mix

In the past, marketing was relevant to only profit-making firms. Recent developments have, however, pushed the social sector to equally adopt marketing precepts. We are, therefore, at a point where there is wide recognition of the importance of marketing to the sustenance of the health service. Marketing essentially refers to the set of well-coordinated activities geared towards the achievement of market needs. The strategic management of this process leaves much more to be gained than lost (Liberman & Rotarius, 2001). It involves the creation, offer, and communication of offerings that satisfy consumer wants in ways leading to repeat purchase. The use of these salient concepts (7Ps) in proportionate forms is critical to the execution of marketing excellence, especially in the health service sector, where goods and services are mainly intangible. Consumers of healthcare constitute a market that is as diverse as a market can be (Calkins & Sviokla, 2007). In view of this reality, there has to be a commensurate combination of these components to allow for an effective and efficient marketing plan. Historically, a marketing plan revolves around the mix of product, price, place, and promotion (McCarthy, 1960). Being a service, this then moves into the domain of the 7Ps; with the additions of physical evidence, people, and process. Here, we will focus extensively on the components of the extended marketing mix (7Ps) as is applicable in the healthcare organization.

### *Healthcare Product*

The health market is fast becoming a more important market in both developing and less developing countries (Zaltman & Vertinsky, 1971). Like in other markets, this market offers products and services directed at the satisfaction and delight of the customer. Products are offerings of value, from a selling entity to a buying entity, at a price. They can be tangible or intangible. As a characteristic of the healthcare sector, these products are more intangible than tangible. Whether tangible or intangible, these components must be combined effectively in a proportionate manner that ultimately will provide quality healthcare. Product offerings must be acceptable to the target recipients for whom they have been created. This target group of people is collectively referred to as customers. Fundamentally, customers are people to whom a service or product is offered at a price. By our earlier assertion, customers are the buying entity. These customers are the lifeblood of every business. Businesses must, therefore, consistently provide offerings/contributions that genuinely meet the unique needs concerning these customers at a price that is commensurate with the quality of the product/service. The basic purpose is to make the customer happy in order to instigate repeat purchase.

The product is the tangible or intangible utility that the customer enjoys, at a price. Product definition enables the match of product qualities (technical, functional, etc.) against the expectations of customers or consumers who patronize these products/services (Kalyanaram & Krishnan, 1997). The product range of the healthcare organization includes but is not limited to consultancy (general or specialist), prescriptions, drugs (injections, oral pills, intravenous solutions), surgical procedures (simple to complex procedures, medical, cosmetic), stay-in facilities (admission beds and other applicable details), and so on. These products form the tangible component of the product range.

Medications form the core of common products in the healthcare organization. These medications come in the form of pills, injections, and so on. These drugs have multifaceted purposes and are directed at a multitude of ailment. While many of them are essentially medical, a few of these products are also used for cosmetic purposes. These products may vary in form, type, and purpose from one place to the other, based on commonly diagnosed ailments and the nature of the services customers seek. In Africa, where there is malaria, it is almost impossible to go to a healthcare center that does not have medications to cure malaria. It is a common ailment in Ghana and so many hospitals and other caregivers have products to curb the disease. Medical product needs vary from place to place and from people to people. Medical practitioners must, therefore, be very knowledgeable of the environment where they operate. This will enable the provision of the desired needed products to satisfy the unique and diverse needs of these customers.

The product in the health sector is primarily and collectively the various offerings available to a customer (patient). Consultancy, drugs and medication, laboratory and diagnostic services, and surgical procedures are some of the products available in the healthcare organization. Apart from the drugs and medications that patients make tangible use of (by swallowing or through injections), a large part of the product range is intangible. Let us make the point clear that, even for the tangible part of the product range, it is difficult to separate the service from the product. The quality of service that accompanies the administration of the physical product, to a considerable extent, determines the ultimate overall satisfaction of the customer (patient) with the physical product. The concept of Product-services is very useful in the healthcare organization.

Consultancy, laboratory, and diagnostic services must be delivered with great quality to make the desired impact. Healthcare is a rather necessary and sensitive need area, which should be handled with sufficient care. Unfortunately, for the same reasons of necessity and sensitivity, customer would seek healthcare, regardless of the quality of the service and many of these customers endure pathetic and sad service delivery cultures. The healthcare system must rise above this and put the customer first. The product offerings, after all, are offered at a price, customers, therefore, deserve their money's worth. This leads us to our next marketing mix element of price.

## Healthcare Price

In many exchange relationships, there is a price element. Medical care comes at a fee and customers are intensely participative in their healthcare decisions as a result of the ever-rising cost of medical care (Corbin, Kelley, & Schwartz, 2001). Healthcare pricing has always been complex. Generally, healthcare service providers do not disclose prices prior to service, and thus, consumers are increasingly concerned and demand price transparency. Advancements in medicine and related fields have increased the price of assessing healthcare in most cases. High cost of research and accompanying resources are all incorporated into the price of medical care. The availability of new research in diagnostics, maternal care, and heart procedures has significantly induced the high price of medical care (Bodenheimer, 2005).

In most places, there are health schemes that are making it easier for patients to afford this rising price of medical care. Many people have died, not because they suffered incurable diseases, no, but because they could not afford the price of simple medical procedures. When this happens, the insensitivity of the healthcare organization is highlighted. The point, however, is this: In the end, the hospital must be able to cover its operational costs and be able to pay its staff, its creditors, and others who are featured on their payroll. How would they do this on the altar of free medical care? Your guess is as good as mine. A workable way to reduce this cost burden is for the state to develop adequate policy measures on health schemes. The state should be able to develop schemes that incorporate adequately the needs of the poor and powerless. People must not be denied medical care because they cannot afford to pay for it. Governments must design social programs that give importance to maximum healthcare for all its citizenry. Governments cannot execute this alone; businesses, well-wishing organizations, nongovernmental organizations, and private individuals must all in one way or the other augment the effort of governments to give premium care to its people. This way, price hikes associated with medical care will become less burdensome for many people. After all that has been said and done, the healthcare organizations must, also for their own sake, price their products and services appropriately to prevent driving away their customers to alternative places. Healthcare organizations must take into consideration the price of similar health organizations, their own cost elements, and other prevailing economic conditions in setting their price. Finally, the customer must derive satisfaction and pleasure that the price they pay to access healthcare is commensurate with average incomes.

## *Healthcare Place*

Place in healthcare refers to the network of locations where customers can seek healthcare. Health centers must be distributed in a manner that makes for easy accessibility. Customers of health are everywhere; it is a need that cuts across race, gender, wealth, and so on. Places of medical care must be adequately communicated, to further increase the ease of accessibility. Incorrect facility location decisions have a serious impact on the community, beyond simply cost and service metrics. For instance, hard-to-access healthcare facilities are likely to be associated with increased morbidity and mortality (Ahmadi-Javid, Seyedi, & Syam, 2017). Healthcare providers are increasingly shifting their focus to ambulatory care—medical services performed on an outpatient basis without admission to a hospital or other facilities. In addition to inpatient care, hospitals are also providing services through outpatient facilities which are conveniently located in underserved areas, easily accessible to patients and medical professionals.

## *Healthcare Promotion*

Usually, healthcare organizations do not pursue marketing communications as robustly as do traditional marketing-oriented businesses. However, whether flamboyant or modest, healthcare places must adequately incorporate promotional tools into their marketing efforts to yield maximum results. Against this background, healthcare centers must take advantage of salient promotional tools to maintain their competitive relevance. Promotion is the key aspect of the healthcare marketing mix, which consists of advertising, personal selling, public relations, and sales promotion. There are many communication modes available to reach the target market of the healthcare organization. For instance, information can be geared towards the ultimate choice of healthier lifestyles (Ling, Franklin, Lindsteadt, & Gearon, 1992). Communications in the healthcare organization, however, must not be ultimately linked to profit motives. Profit is important, but this is the sector where social marketing rather than anything else is needed.

Markets globally experience wide and varying degrees of health issues, thus, increasing the need for social marketing. Social marketing uses socially acceptable marketing precepts to cause positive changes in behavior and to promote public health (Grier & Bryant, 2005). This approach has grown in popularity and usage and is an effective way to change health behavior and improve health, both at the individual level and at the wider societal level. The healthcare organization must target behavioral change in its promotional efforts. Free screening activities, health talks, and many other health services and mediums will cause the desired social change we need in terms of keeping healthy. At the same time, there are communication media to promote these healthcare organizations. The next time somebody you screened for free is unwell/sick, they may want to come to your facility again to access care and that is the essence of marketing communications.

### Healthcare People

People refer fundamentally to the human elements who work to deliver the mandate of the organization. In the healthcare organization, just like in other service sectors, people are an essential component of service delivery. Proper management of the workforce is critical in improving the quality of services and health outcomes. Medical officers and other employees of health centers must be sympathetic to the needs of their customers and deliver this crucial service softly and with gentle care. The patience and maturity of a nurse contribute significantly to offering that calm restoration every ailing person requires. The willingness and ability of a medical officer to provide relevant explanations to a patient's questions and worries build trust and give hope to a dying patient. The concept of relationship marketing has become vital in delivering the service mandate. Many organizations are interested in establishing valuable relationships with their customers. People working in healthcare organizations must endeavour to develop relationships that make the exchange process valuable to the customer.

### Healthcare Process

The process by which healthcare service is delivered is complicated, as it involves a complex system, human activities, and real-time decision-making. Processes leading up to the receipt of medical care must be simplified to the barest minimum to make easy access to the service. Health information systems that compile, manage, store, and transmit healthcare data can be useful in improving the service delivery process. Cumbersome registration and billing procedures only make the patient sicker. Information technology can be beneficial in improving the quality, safety, and efficiency of healthcare. The healthcare organization must automate their processes and procedures to make them less cumbersome.

### Healthcare Physical Evidence

Hospitals and medical centers are not pleasant places for anybody to visit. These places must, therefore, exhibit some physical characteristics that make it easier and more comfortable for customers. This is known as physical evidence. What would make you choose one medical facility over the other? Commonly, patients want to see a clean structure; clean bathrooms that smell right, a well-kept reception area with comfortable waiting area facilities, smart-looking medical officers, clean bedding for in-house treatment, laboratory and surgical centers with relevant diagnostic tools/machines, and pharmaceutical sections. Patients value the built environment of hospital facilities that offers a homely and welcoming atmosphere, a supportive environment, a functional physical design, access to external areas, and provision of facilities for recreation and leisure (Douglas & Douglas, 2004). Physical evidence influences patients' satisfaction, perceived service quality, and loyalty. For example, the hospital atmosphere has a significant relationship with patient-perceived outcomes (Narang, Ritu, Polsa, Soneye, & Fuxiang, 2015).

## Conclusion

Variations in common attributes, routines, and other population features are all adding up to facilitate the rising importance of healthcare marketing. Some tendencies in the healthcare field are predicted to continue in the future. From the 1970s, the healthcare terrain has gradually changed from medical care toward healthcare. The rising knowledge of the link between health status and lifestyle has incited a switch from a strictly medical model of health and illness to that which imbibes more of a social and psychological standpoint. This has incited a switch from a sternly medical model of health and illness to that which imbibes more of a social and psychological standpoint.

Thomas (2004) postulates that marketing in healthcare in the 21st century is a true reflection of the industry as well as the society it is found in, just like the case of the mold and domain of healthcare. Like other institutions, it surfaces in the society it finds itself in, hence, it tries to meet the expectations of the people of the society in that particular geographical region. Different processes have been put in place to make sure the well-being of people is assured in every society. Healthcare has become a defying sector that is very significant in every developed or developing nations of the world.

The 20th century revolution in culture, put a spotlight on the value healthcare professionals deliver to customers in the process of rendering services to them. This built a strong foundation for the healthcare institution, even with the increasing trends in factors such as successes clocked in economies of countries, educational improvements, and scientific and technological progress. Demographic trends have also affected the healthcare institution in terms of age structure, household and family structure, and consumer attitudes. Different lifestyles revolving around these trends have made the 21st-century consumer more dynamic and demanding, thereby, putting clinicians and managers on their toes to gain loyalty from these consumers and achieve customer equity with them. This has pushed many healthcare institutions to develop processes that give them competitive advantages in their growing industry. The fact remains, with the term patient being increasingly pushed aside in preference for the word consumer, there is a call for a notable move in the way healthcare organizations structure their marketing strategies. This has given the receiver of healthcare the upper hand in recent times to dictate the processes chosen by healthcare institutions.

## Review Questions

1. Identify three key demographic factors and elaborate on their impact on the evolution of healthcare.
2. Outline and explain four key developments in healthcare in the 21st century.
3. Identify three key factors affecting the adoption of marketing in healthcare.
4. List and explain the components of the marketing mix applicable in a healthcare organization.

### MINI CASE STUDY: HEALTHCARE PRICING

Susan J. Patrick had a toothache. Years earlier, she had a root canal procedure, but could not afford to have the tooth crowned, which would have assured complete recovery. She made an appointment with the privately owned Bazo Dental Clinic in Lufasi, Ghana. The clinic had an inviting, attractive service-scape—the *physical environment*. The front desk staff made her feel welcome and comfortable. After filling out a brief questionnaire about her health history, she was directed to a well-appointed waiting area that offered bottled water and current magazine selections.

That comfort level changed when she met the dentist, Dr. Ajololo. He examined the tooth, then told her that it would cost GH900 cedis to have the tooth crowned and that it would have to be carried out soon or she would lose her tooth. Susan was alarmed by his brusque tone. He offered neither comfort nor explanation about the procedure.

Because Susan was unable to afford to pay such a large bill, she asked about payment plans. The doctor turned away from her and, as he left the room, told the nurse to inform her that Bazo Clinic does not have payment plans. Susan paid the minimal consultation fee, then left unhappy at the thought that, without the crown, she would lose her tooth in less than a week. She told her friend about her experience, and her friend recommended Cliff Dental Clinic. There, Susan found that though the servicescape was not quite as elegant as the Bazo Clinic, the staff were friendly and helpful. The new crown cost far less, GH500 cedis, and she was able to pay it off in three monthly payments. Susan saved her tooth as well as her money, and she was happy. She became an advocate for the Cliff Dental Clinic and shared her bad experience at the Bazo Clinic with her family and friends.

**Discussion Questions**

1. Do you think Susan would have gone ahead with the procedure at Bazo Dental Clinic if there was a payment plan, regardless of how she was attended to by Dr. Ajololo? Explain your answer.
2. Cliff Dental Clinic carried out the same procedure at GHC500, GHC400 less than the price at Bazo Clinic. Is it fair to conclude that the Bazo Clinic offers higher quality dental care service than Cliff Clinic? What factors may have played into the difference in the price?
3. Bazo Clinic does not offer payment plans. What other arrangements do you suggest Bazo Clinic should put in place to make pricing attractive and affordable to its target market?

# References

Ahmadi-Javid, A., Seyedi, P., & Siddhartha, S. S. (2017). A survey of healthcare facility location. *Computers & Operations Research, 79*, 223–263.

Andaleeb, S. S. (2001). Service quality perceptions and patient satisfaction: a study of hospitals in a developing country. *Social Science & Medicine, 52*(9), 1359–1370.

Basics for Health. (2018, April 16). *Social determinants of health.* Retrieved from http://www.basicsforhealthsociety.ca/

Beaupert, F., Carney, T., Chiarella, M., Satchell, C., Walton, M., Bennett, B., & Kelly, P. (2014). Regulating healthcare complaints: A literature review. *International Journal of Healthcare Quality Assurance, 27*(6), 505–518.

Betancourt, J. R., Green, A. R., & Carrillo, J. E. (2002). *Cultural competence in health care: Emerging frameworks and practical approaches.* New York, NY: Commonwealth Fund.

Black, N. (2013). Patient reported outcome measures could help transform healthcare. *BMJ, 346,* f167.

Boonekamp, L. C. (1994). Emerald article: Marketing for health-care organizations: An introduction to network management. *Medicine, 8*(5), 11–24.

Bodenheimer, T. (2005). High and rising health care costs. Part 2: technologic innovation. *Annals of Internal Medicine, 142*(11), 932–937.

Boutayeb, A., & Boutayeb, S. (2005). The burden of non-communicable diseases in developing countries. *International Journal for Equity in Health, 4*(2). https://doi.org/10.1186/1475-9276-4-2

Bowden, D. E., & Smits, S. J. (2012). Managing in the context of healthcare's escalating technology and evolving culture. *Journal of Health Organization and Management, 26*(2), 149–157.

Bramlett, M. D., & Blumberg, S. J. (2007). Family structure and children's physical and mental health. *Health Affairs, 26*(2), 549–558.

Breton, M., Lamothe, L., & Denis, J. L. (2014) How organizations can act as institutional entrepreneurs in a context of change. *Journal of Health Organization and Management, 28*(1), 77–95.

Calkins, C., & Sviokla, J. (2007). What health consumers want. *Harvard Business Review, 85*(12), 14–15.

Corbin, C. L., Kelley, S. W., & Schwartz, R. W. (2001). Concepts in service marketing for healthcare professionals. *The American Journal of Surgery, 181*(1), 1–7.

Crepaldi, C., De Rosa, E., & Pesce, F. (2012). *Literature review on innovation in social services in Europe* (sectors of Health, Education and Welfare Services). Report. IRS.

Dell'Aversana, G., & Bruno, A. (2017). Different and similar at the same time. Cultural Competence through the leans of healthcare providers. *Frontiers in Psychology, 8,* 1–6.

Douglas, C. H., & Douglas, M. R. (2004). Patient-friendly hospital environments: Exploring the patients' perspective. *Health Expectations, 7*(1), 61–73.

Escarce, J. J., & Kapur, K. (2006). Access to and quality of health care. In M. Tienda & F. Mitchell (Eds.), *Hispanics and the future of America* (pp. 410–446). Washington, DC: National Academies Press.

Frambach, R. T., Wels-Lips, I., & Gündlach, A. (1997). Proactive product service strategies: an application in the European health market. *Industrial Marketing Management, 26*(4), 341–352.

Gambarov, V., Sarno, D., Hysa, X., Calabrese, M., & Bilotta, A. (2017). The role of loyalty programs in healthcare service ecosystems. *The TQM Journal, 29*(6), 899–919.

Gould, S. J. (2018). Consumer attitudes toward health and healthcare: A differential perspective. *Journal of Consumer Affairs, 22*(1), 96–118.

Grier, S., & Bryant, C. A. (2005). Social marketing in public health. *Annual Review of Public Health, 26,* 319–339.

Hayden, V. (1993). How to increase market orientation. *Journal of Management in Medicine, 7*(1), 29–46.

Jarvis, L. C. (2016). Shame and institutional stability or change in healthcare. *International Journal of Sociology and Social Policy, 36*(3/4), 173–189.

Kalyanaram, G., & Krishnan, V. (1997). Deliberate product definition: Customizing the product definition process. *Journal of Marketing Research, 34*(2), 276–285.

Liberman, A., & Rotarius, T. M. (2001). Marketing in today's health care environment. *The health care manager, 19*(4), 23–28.

Light, D. W. (2002). Institutional change and healthcare organizations: From professional dominance to managed care. *International Journal of Integrated Care, 2*(1), 1–2.

Ling, J. C., Franklin, B. A., Lindsteadt, J. F., & Gearon, S. A. (1992). Social marketing: its place in public health. *Annual Review of Public Health, 13*(1), 341–362.

Longo, D. R., Land, G., & Wayne Schramm, W. (1997). Consumer reports in healthcare Do they make a difference in patient care? *AMA Journal of Ethics, 278*(19), 1579–1584.

McCarthy, E. J. (1960). *Basic marketing: A managerial approach.* Homewood, IL: Irwin.

Mesabbah, M., & Arisha, A. (2016). Performance management of the public healthcare services in Ireland a review. *International Journal of Healthcare Quality Assurance, 29*(2), 209–235.

Mohrman, S. A., & Shani, A. B. (2014) Healthcare: An ecosystem in transition. Reconfiguring the ecosystem for sustainable healthcare. *Organizing for Sustainable Effectiveness, 4,* 1–29.

Morgan, B. (2018, January 9). *The top 5 trends in customer experience for healthcare.* Retrieved from https://www.forbes.com/sites/blakemorgan/2018/01/09/the-top-5-trends-in-customer-experience-for-healthcare/

Narang, R., Polsa, P., Soneye, A., & Fuxiang, W. (2015). Impact of hospital atmosphere on perceived health care outcome. *International Journal of Health Care Quality Assurance, 28*(2), 129–140. https://doi.org/10.1108/IJHCQA-12-2013-0142

Nordin, P., Kork, A. A., & Koskela, I. (2017). Value-based healthcare measurement as a context for organizational learning: Adding a strategic edge to assess health outcome. *Leadership in Health Services, 30*(2), 159–170.

Porter, M. E. (2010). What is value in health care? *New England Journal of Medicine, 363*(26), 2477–2481.

Sheingold, B. H., & Hahn, J. A. (2014). The history of healthcare quality: The first 100 years 1860–1960. *International Journal of African Nursing Sciences, 1,* 18–22.

Shi, L., & Singh, D. A. (2017). *Delivering health care in America: A systems approach* (7th ed.). Burlington, MA: Jones & Bartlett Learning.

Te Ara Encyclopedia of New Zealand. (2018, April 16). *Health and society.* Retrieved from https://teara.govt.nz/en/health-and-society

Thomas, R. K. (2004). *Marketing health services. The evolving societal and healthcare context.* Chicago, IL: Health Administration Press.

Torrens, P. R. (1993). Historical evolution and overview of health services in the United States. In S. J. Williams & P. R. Torrens (Eds.), *Introduction to health services* (4th ed.; pp. 4–30). New York, NY: Wiley.

Utica College. (2018, April 14). *9 new trends in healthcare management for 2017.* Retrieved from https://programs.online.utica.edu/articles/10-trends-in-health-care-management-0321

von Eiff, W. (2015). International benchmarking and best practice management: In search of healthcare and hospital excellence. In S. C. Buttigieg, C. Rathert, & W. Von Eiff (Eds.), *International best practices in healthcare management* (pp. 223–252). Bradford, England: Emerald Group.

Zaltman, G., & Vertinsky, I. (1971). Health service marketing: a suggested model. *Journal of Marketing, 35*(3), 19–27.

# 4

## Public Sector Marketing in Healthcare

### Chapter Outline

- Introduction
- Key Characteristics of Public Services
- Scope and Nature of Public Sector Marketing
- Importance of Marketing in the Public Sector
- Challenges of Public Sector Marketing
- The Marketing Mix of Public Sector Marketing
- Types of Marketing in the Public Sector
- Social Marketing
- Aspects of Social Marketing
- The Public Sector Marketing Planning Process
- Conclusion
- Review Questions
- Mini Case Study With Discussion Questions
- References

*Marketing in Healthcare-Related Industries*, pages 77–104
Copyright © 2020 by Information Age Publishing
All rights of reproduction in any form reserved.

## Chapter Outcome

By the end of this chapter, the reader will be able to

- understand the concept of public sector marketing,
- identify the role of the 7Ps of services marketing in public sector marketing,
- identify the importance of public sector marketing, and
- understand the major challenges of public sector marketing.

## Introduction

This chapter is an introduction to the fundamentals and concepts of public sector marketing. Governments (public sector entities) are involved in the healthcare sector in many ways. From large public hospitals to ministries of health, through national health services to HIV aid commissions, there are several ways by which the public sector engages in the delivery of health services all over the world. Public sector marketing, however, takes on a different course because unlike the private sector, profit is not always the overriding concern in the delivery of public sector health services. Government provision is generally believed to be less technically efficient than private provision, and medical care is no exception. However, a lack of a profit motive may be a virtue in some cases. While private providers may not act in the public interest (e.g., a for-profit hospital that skimps on medical care because skimping is hard to detect), government provision may be superior to private sector provision.

This chapter is devoted to exploring the nuances of public sector marketing. In this chapter, there will be a focus on the challenges and importance of public sector marketing. Additionally, the concept of social marketing and its function in public sector marketing will be explained. This chapter covers issues such as the characteristics of public services, scope, and nature of public sector marketing; how public sector marketing differs from other forms of marketing; the 7Ps of services marketing; social marketing; the need for public sector marketing; and challenges of public sector marketing.

## Key Characteristics of Public Services

According to Graham (1994), there is a widespread acceptance that one of the main attributes of the public goods and services is that, the fundamental reason behind their provision cannot be framed simply in economic terms. Wherefore, economic considerations in the private sector such as efficiency and profitability, ascertain decision-making in democratic nations. These decision pertain to social justice, equity, and legitimacy. These are notionally preeminent in the public sector. Given the centrality of noneconomic objectives of public services, the usage of traditional economic-based performance measures at the operational level is inappropriate within the increasingly managerialist culture. According to Bauer (1966), these necessitate the use of wider social indicators for evaluating performance at the strategic level. One of the profits that accrue to the delivery of public service is social profit or social capital. For instance, the improvements in the health status of the population and the levels of educational attainment are some of the profits.

Moreover, the connection between the people who use the public service and the public services themselves has been defined historically concerning citizenship rather than consumerism. Consequently, there is a perception that the order of service usage and attitude with regards to public service vary significantly from private service. According to Scrivens (1991), this varies by requiring a reframing of present models of consumer behavior. It is debated that the primary concept of citizenship is underscored by a collectivist philosophy. This philosophy places emphasis on the wider needs of social justice and the needs of the society rather than the narrow needs of the individual. It, therefore, highlights the responsibilities and the rights of the citizens. There is an emphasis on the equality of all citizens within such a concept, and afterwards, the relevance of the citizens' equal rights to have access to services regardless of the ability to pay. Nevertheless, there is growing stress on the individual consumer and the associated demands for customer-focused service provision. This highlights one of the essential issues the public service faces. Some of these issues or problems include defining and identifying the public service customer.

In addition to what has been mentioned above, there is a rising concern that the concept of customers in public service is multidimensional and complex. This highlights two core characteristics of public services. These are, individual and social benefits involved, and the payment and consumption of such services. In clear terms, there are multiple beneficiaries in many public services. These include education and social care. These beneficiaries include individual service recipients, and also incorporates the service recipient's family, the service recipient's employer, and may legitimately consider the customer as well as society. This is complicated further by the existence of an indirect payment receipt. This relates to many services, such as bringing firms that disburse public money and individual taxpayers into the equation as extra prospective customers.

In the healthcare context, social justice may be defined as equality in access to and quality of healthcare and the right to health for everyone (Wilkinson, 1996). Health is of particular importance to society and to all members in a society, regardless of social status. Members/citizens should be able to have access to affordable, adequate, and quality healthcare in a fair and equitable manner (Braveman et al., 2011). However, there is substantial evidence for racial/ethnic disparities in health-related lifestyles and health status, exhibiting the need for social justice in all areas of the public's healthcare. For example, older minority Americans, particularly African Americans, experience worse health conditions and have shorter life expectancies than majority groups. Research shows that the rates of losing health insurance coverage are higher among African Americans and Hispanic young men and women and this remains high throughout adulthood, which may contribute to biases in referrals to specialists and in receiving surgical procedures (Einbinder & Schulman, 2000; Sohn, 2017). Similarly, rural residents, regardless of race and ethnicity, have lower levels of insurance coverage. The homeless have a very high prevalence of untreated conditions.

## Scope and Nature of Public Sector Marketing

Marketing as a discipline was born and developed primarily in the private sector. It was initially seen as relating to fast-moving consumer goods and only in the 1980s was its application in the public sector considered. Kotler and Levy (1969) were the forerunners of the move towards broadening the scope of marketing. The scholars debated that every firm has to concentrate on customers whose needs can be recognized and fulfilled through the operative application of marketing practices. As such, marketing abilities in effectively advancing this process should make it applicable, notwithstanding whether the organization is in the public or private sector. In an era where public sector organizations must perform better in response to the public interest, whether they are in charge of governance or producing goods and services, marketing can help.

Marketing represents a blend of management tasks and decisions directed at meeting the opportunities and threats in the changing marketing environment. Marketing aims at providing market offerings that satisfy consumers' needs and wants, so that the objectives of the enterprise, as of the consumer and society are achieved. The core notions of marketing, therefore, are satisfaction and exchange. A business that adopts the marketing approach endeavors to create exchanges with the consumer in mind. This enables the business to achieve its goal of profits, and the consumer to also achieve his or her goal of satisfaction and value for money. Government organizations can engage in marketing according to this definition. For instance, when a government institution develops a product or service, be it a physical product, an idea such as "don't smoke in public," or the provision of a service such as the maintenance of a national park for visitors, the institution prices, promotes, and distributes it to a targeted audience to create an exchange. In this case, marketing has taken place.

Among public sector professionals, the concept of marketing has widely been perceived as an obviously commercial concept clothed in a populist transactional guise. This is with regards to both the origin of and the significance to public sector firms that are concerned with the conveyance of "public-good" services (Caruana, Ramaseshan, & Ewing, 1997; Walsh, 1991). Therefore, marketing has been perceived by these scholars as the worst, most irrelevant, and conflicting means of conveying services to the public (Laing & McKee, 2001).

One of the major reasons for the continued confusion over marketing application in this area is the sheer diversity of organizations covered by the "public sector." Whereas it is easy to see marketing's application in some of the large public institutions, it is problematic when a local authority department is considered. As a result, marketing in public sector institutions is largely a piecemeal and reactive, rather than an integrated and proactive undertaking/approach where it can generate the most synergy. The work of the public sector has major implications for economies, since the relevance, efficiency, effectiveness, sustainability, and impact of a country's public sector is vital to national welfare and its organizations (Laing, 2003). Additionally, managerialism over the last decade has grown, and marketing has begun to attract more widespread attention, especially in relation to core public services such as health and education (Walsh, 1991). Increasingly, the lines between the private sector and the public sector models are blurring; managers should not regard the private-public context as a dichotomy, but rather as a continuum from "pure private" to "pure public" (Laing, 2003).

The public sector deals with the production, delivery, and allocation of basic public goods and services at global, national, regional, and local levels. Its processes and structures take the form of direct administration, public corporations, and partial outsourcing. Its activities are funded through government expenditure and financed by seigniorage, taxes, and government borrowing or through grants. Most public goods at the most basic level are services other than physical products. The unique attributes of services include perishability, intangibility, heterogeneity, and inseparability (Zeithaml, Parasuraman, & Berry, 1985). Nevertheless, going beyond this basic level, the key characteristics of the public services are partitioned into three categories. These three categories include the relevance of the citizen other than the consumer and the dominance of political objectives other than that of economic objectives. Based on the perspectives of Lovelock and Weinberg (1990), the last characteristics of the public services include the need to serve several multidimensional consumers and customers.

## Importance of Marketing in the Public Sector

The rise and increasing role of the public services within the economy have been acknowledged as very important to the services of the public. It is, therefore, important for public firms to acquire distinct skills, favorable image, and services adapted to customer needs. To start with, marketing in the public sector, in general, helps to see customers as citizens. The role of the public sector helps to build long term relationships with the government and customers as well. Public sector marketing, according to Kotler and Levy (1969), helps the government to supply two types of products. The first one is a physical product. This type of product can be exchanged directly. The second type of product is called the *idea* product. This type of product is the type that paves the way for the government to sell their political actions by selling their ideas to the public. Literature has demonstrated that these products of public service have become the responsibility of the government to satisfy customer–voter needs. Walsh (1994) maintains that the development of marketing in the public sector is justified so far as it provides sets of instruments that can be used to develop the efficacy and responsiveness of the public service.

Grigorescu (2006) argues that both public and private sector partnership can result in citizen satisfaction and employee's satisfaction. Caruana, Ramaseshan, and Ewing (1997) further assert that in order for the government to accomplish its objectives with regards to accountability and transparency, they need a market orientation. This means that the government needs to apply the marketing concept effectively (Caruana, 2003). Market orientation can also lead to increased performance. Studies have confirmed that there are positive relationships between market orientation and overall performance of public services firms (Caruana & Calleya, 1998; Cervera, Mollá, & Sanchez, 2001). Public marketing is essential in the public sector. This is because it helps to create both customer loyalty and attract new ones, and it also helps entities positioning themselves in a new market. Also, the importance of public sector marketing includes its pricing policy and satisfaction of internal clients. It also includes how public sector marketing integrates the mix of services to satisfy existing and new clients

sector may have limited effect on the introduction of new products. An instance is a treaty to establish a constitution for Europe (TCE). This is commonly referred to as European constitution, which was signed in 2004 by representatives of the 27 European Union (EU) member states, subject to subsequent endorsement.

A well-chosen price in private firms helps them to achieve the financial objectives of the firms. However, the principles of pricing in the private sector cannot be applied to that of the public sector. The public sector is managed as a nonprofit organization, and although a certain surplus may be generated in one period, there is no goal to maximize this surplus in any way. Again, the concept of the readiness to pay for a product can frequently not be applied to the services within the public sector. This is because consumption may not be within the free choice of the customer. Finally, many public sector services do not have any direct competition, so there may be no way to assess the product's positioning. Peattie (2003) maintains that these do not mean that pricing is irrelevant in the public sector, where the services provided are for free. Evidently, there are some situations where asking citizens to pay a price for services become unethical. This is attributed to the fact that the associated costs need to be covered by national and local taxes. In other situations, too, the public sector may intentionally decide to charge for certain services. This is to make them appear more valuable for the consumers (citizen). For instance, in Germany, the prices for the disposal of personal waste rose steadily in the 1980s, which led to an increase in environmental awareness.

Another challenge facing the public sector is perceived price unfairness. The public sector could excessively charge high prices for every service without facing any direct competition from private firms. Besides, the perspective of Xia and Monroe (2004) confirm that citizens may unlikely accept such unfair pricing and may go to the extreme of raising their voices in the form of peaceful demonstrations or stop the consumptions of such services. This, ultimately, creates costs for the public sector. In other severe cases, the citizens may decide to travel to other advanced countries with a more favorable pricing structure. For instance, in the EU, several firms moved their businesses to Ireland, where they had low corporate tax. In addition, it must be stressed also that it may be difficult sometimes to eliminate price unfairness in the public sector. Lamb (1987), argues that one objective of the public sector pricing is income redistribution. This implies that setting prices in the public sector may be different, depending on the situation of the benefiting citizen.

Public expectation of fairness may also mean that every consumer (citizen) should be accorded fair treatment; the same quality of services irrespective of whoever they are and wherever the consumers are. Sometimes, governments tend to spend too much on providing particular services due to their ignorance of how much to invest. This makes the public sector suffer, resulting in high cost. This can further hinder the success of marketing in the public sector. Furthermore, another challenge in the public sector is the low return on investment. This is because selling is not necessarily linked with buying, as recipients do not always have to pay for the product. Also, due to a lack of return on investment and intense competition, it does not force governments to produce products that meet the satisfaction of the customers (citizen). Finally, government and public sector firms that typically have not integrated marketing activities suffer from poor coordination.

## The Marketing Mix of Public Sector Marketing

In this subsection, the focus is on the marketing mix variables used in public sector marketing and how these variables are blended to achieve the overall marketing goals of the public sector. The marketing mix has dominated marketing thought, research, and practice. McCarthy (1960) was the first to offer the marketing mix concept, and it alluded to the product, price, place, and promotion, which was christened the 4Ps of marketing, as a way of translating marketing planning into practice. The marketing mix is anything but a scientific theory that merely acts as a conceptual model for shaping an organization's offerings to suit consumers' needs.

It is rather a necessary component of an organization's strategy for the completion of the objectives of the company. The actual 4Ps of the marketing mix were, however, considered by many to be restrictive, particularly with the advent of the service industry. Bitner and Booms (1981) extended the 4Ps concepts to include three additional Ps, namely, people, physical evidence, and process, to make it 7Ps. The 7Ps are also referred to as the expanded marketing mix, and it recognizes that at the points of service creation and delivery (i.e., service encounters), marketing and operational functions occur simultaneously. The elements within the marketing mix all affect the effectiveness of one another. Marketing mix is successful when the combination of its variables leads to the attainment of organizational objectives.

Effective management of the elements of the marketing mix is instrumental in creating stakeholder value. This is achieved by recognizing that the stakeholders of organizations have different characteristics and, hence, fall under different segments of the market. For this reason, they respond to marketing activities differently. A single marketing strategy may not work for these different stakeholders; different marketing strategies should, therefore, be used for different stakeholders. In other words, the marketing mixes for the various stakeholder groups should be different. Different stakeholder groups have to be targeted, and in turn, the service must be positioned in their minds in such a way that it will be perceived to create value for them.

## Product

The product is actually the services to be provided by the public institution, and it varies from one institution to another. Public institutions use their services as a vehicle to meet the needs of their clients or the general public. It is important to distinguish between what the public institution offers and what benefits consumers derive from these offers. The aim is to ensure that the citizenry gets good services that offer them value for their money. Bagozzi (1975) posits that great service and good value for money will help build long-term relationship. The product idea is based on offering goods and services that are of value to consumers. In a nutshell, the product policy in the public sector pertains to safety, credibility, security, and continuity in values which are in the national interest or in the interest of the greater majority. The quality and quantity of the service are of fundamental importance as these can affect the level of demand for that service and the position of the firm compared to its competitors. To deliver quality service, public sector institutions need to look into the accuracy and reliability of cost figures given in the feasibility studies.

## Price

Price is the fees charged to customers by firms. According to Zeithaml (1988), from the customer's viewpoint, price is what is given up or sacrificed to obtain a product. Firms in the public sector need to have a precise scale of fees for their clients. The fees charged will be higher for a prestige service compared with a standard service. With increasing competition, firms are now more cautious in setting their fees. In the public sector, price is related to the achievement of the government's goals and policies. Pricing is key to a company's profitability and survival. However, in the public sector, pricing decisions present a dilemma between the covering of the cost and the reaction of the people to the rise in price.

Nevertheless, customers in the public sector have to comply with the prices of companies whose services are monopolized. Government agencies are often not responsive to the public because of their monopoly status. The public service sector is usually an outlet through which the government makes profits or satisfy some needs of the citizenry. This makes it difficult for consumers to dispute the pricing policies of public service organizations. To get consumers to purchase an offering, organizations operating in the public sector must ensure that perceived costs in acquiring the firm's offer do not exceed perceived benefits from the perspective of the customer. The consumer is more likely to desist from buying a market offer if the perceived value is low (Kotler & Zaltman, 1971; Weinreich, 2003). Also, free or low-priced products might be perceived as lacking quality, or the beneficiary might not value it or thus feel patronized.

## Place

Place refers to the location where a product or service can be obtained or purchased by consumers. Firms need to be concerned with how accessible their services are to their clients. Channels are designed by firms to distribute their products and services to their clients and should be convenient to the clients. According to Bruce (1998), distribution involves a series of activities to ensure that products get to customers when and wherever they want them. When the market offering is good, distribution channels that are appropriate, ample, and compatible should be used (Kotler & Zaltman, 1971). Government and public sector organizations, thus, need to ensure that their offerings can be conveniently accessed by consumers.

The target market of the public sector is represented with dispersed consumers, and a number of place or distribution variations may be required when the target markets are dispersed or have different needs. The distribution channel has to respond to the mission of the particular public service. This means finding a balance in delivering the service to all citizens without reducing accessibility. This is especially important concerning individuals who are disabled or have to overcome language barriers (Shapiro, 1973). That is why the National Health Service (NHS) relies on intensive distribution. It aims to make the provision of its services convenient to citizens by engaging in continuous and mass distribution via conferences and workshops (Sheaff, 1991).

## Promotion

The objective of promotion is to communicate or sell a firm's goods and services by informing, persuading, and reminding the target market and audience about the availability of the good or service and its benefits. This can be done through the various forms of promotional mix: personal selling, advertising, publicity, public relations, and so on. With respect to firms that decide to advertise, they will need to draw up an advertising program to meet the professional requirements and at the same time, portray the firm's desired corporate image. In order to create and sustain the demand for an offering, its benefits have to be communicated to the clients repeatedly to attain the top of mind awareness. Communications represent the process of transmitting messages to make the organizations' products or services attractive to the target customer. Therefore, the communication of the image of public service has an impact on the consumer's perceived values of the government policy. The principles and methods of communicating promotional messages to consumers are also, in essence, the same as those in the commercial markets, although the message content is likely to differ.

## *People*

The service personnel are the people who provide the firm's services to its clients. They are very important due to the difficulty in separating them from the service offering. They, therefore, symbolize the image of the firm by how they behave and act. All the marketing efforts undertaken to attract customers can be a waste, if the service personnel fail to treat customers right by being cold or rude. In contrast, the warm or friendly nature of service personnel can increase customer satisfaction and retention, thereby, leading to customer loyalty (Kotler, 1982). The employees need to be well trained in customer service, and all of them must realize that their own job satisfaction ultimately rests on the success of the organization. Clients' perceptions of the quality of services can also be influenced by other clients. There are a few ways in which firms may maintain and improve the quality of their personnel as well as their performance. These include:

- careful selection and training of personnel,
- activating an awareness towards marketing within the organization,
- ensuring consistent physical appearance, and
- careful control through an internal service personnel audit.

## *Physical Evidence*

Physical evidence influences customers' perception of the service deliverer. It describes the environment and atmosphere where service encounters occur. Physical evidence consists of the physical environment, the facilitating goods that enable the services to be performed and other tangible clues. Managing physical evidence is imperative because consumers perceive the image of the firm through its physical environment and facilitating goods. However, the image of a firm can be difficult to define, measure, and control, because consumer perception about it is subjective. Firms, nonetheless, have the opportunity of managing physical evidence in a way that the desired image conforms to the perceived image.

## *Process*

Processes are an integral part of the production, administration, and the marketing functions of firms. The interest of clients goes beyond the end results of service encounters to the processes by which the services of firms are delivered. Customers tend to judge services by the efficiency and effectiveness of the service process. This is determined by the following: the policies and procedures adopted, the degree of mechanization applied in the provision of service, the level of discretion exhibited by service staff, the extent to which the customer is involved in the service performance, the length of time the consumer has to wait, the flow of information and service, and the available capacity levels.

## Types of Marketing in the Public Sector

Most government sector organizations perceive that marketing is for privately owned ventures whose major mandate is profit-making. This is due to a lack of understanding of the different types of marketing they can undertake. Resultantly, several public sector firms have failed to market effectively. Although public sector marketing is often portrayed as a monolith, marketing in the government sector is quite different. The main forms of marketing that occur in public institutions can be seen in a typology of four different branches of marketing.

## *Marketing of Products and Services*

Surprisingly, the marketing of products and services such as statistical information is the first type of marketing that governmental firms engage in. It is essential to stress that products and services marketed in the government sector are similar to those products and services in the private sector. An example is what the Certified Hospitality Supervisor (CHS) experience illustrates. The CHS is responsible for the oceans and waterways in Canada. With CHS, legislation obligates recreational mariners and commercial mariners to do business in unknown waterways to transport according to certified charts. In order to fulfill the requirement of the legislation, CHS sells electronic and paper charts to recreational boaters and commercial mariners, among others. These recreational boaters and commercial mariners make use of Canada's oceans and waterways. The charts of the CHS concentrate on its marketing objectives. These include designing, developing, and then producing a wide range of products (tide tables, paper and electronic charts, etc.) and CHS also distributes products through systems of distributors in Canada. The marketing objectives further involve pricing and promoting various products in various ways so as to get them to the attention of consumers. In recent times, the adoption of a marketing approach by CHS helped to better meet the needs of its consumers (Canadian mariner community) in order to attain its revenue targets. The CHS has formalized its marketing in diverse ways, which include the following:

- establishing a marketing group to lead its cross-Canada marketing initiatives;
- administering marketing training, education, and research; and
- bringing out a formal marketing strategy to drive future decision making.

### Policy Marketing

Policy marketing is the third type of marketing that governments engage in. Typically, this happens when governments introduce marketing programs aimed at convincing people in particular sectors of society to consent to specific government policies that affect them. For example, when the government attempted to convince the public of the benefits of the Value Added Tax in Ghana, it was engaging in policy marketing. Policy marketing by governments is mostly like "advocacy advertising" by private companies, that is, companies advocating their virtues as good corporate citizens.

### Demarketing or Don't-Use-Our-Programs Marketing

Demarketing refers to campaigns embarked by governments to advise and persuade the target audience to desist from using government programs which were available to them previously. Demarketing has existed for so many years, and in recent times, the concept advanced in tandem with downsizing activities. For instance, several community-based organizations that used to receive funding from government departments in times past have witnessed a substantial decrease in such funds. To mitigate the effects of this on the community-based organizations, departments provide marketing training for the staff of the organizations affected to assist them in establishing an alternative fund base. Demarketing would be relevant in the case of a public sector hospital that wanted to downsize its staff and use more technology (like artificial intelligence, etc.) to become more efficient and deliver better value to its patients.

### Social Marketing

Social marketing is defined as the design, implementation, and control of programs calculated to influence the acceptability of social ideas and involves consideration of product planning, pricing, communication, distribution, and marketing research (Kotler & Zaltman, 1971, p. 5). The most common type of social marketing practiced by governmental firms seeks to change the attitudes and behaviors of targeted groups. For instance, when the Electricity Company of Ghana (ECG) developed the campaign encouraging electricity consumers to use energy-saving bulbs and to take more responsibility for their household energy consumption, it was engaging in social marketing. Similarly, the Ghana Health Service is engaging in social marketing when it develops an advertising campaign intended to persuade young Ghanaians not to begin smoking. Social marketing plays less significant roles in private sector marketing as compared to mainstream or traditional marketing of goods and services.

Social marketing is the application of marketing concepts, techniques, and knowledge to enhance social issues along with economic goals. It encompasses the analysis of social steps of marketing policies, decisions, and activities (Lazer & Kelley, 1973). Andreasen (1993) also defined social marketing as the application of commercial marketing technologies to the analysis, planning, execution, and evaluation of programs designed to influence the voluntary behavior of target audiences in order to improve their personal welfare and that of their society. In addition, French and Blair-Stevens (2006) defined social marketing as the logical application of marketing in conjunction with other concepts and techniques to achieve specific behavioral goals for social or public good.

From the various definitions, social marketing practices are steered by ethical values and seek to integrate research, best practice, theory, audience, and partnership insight to inform the delivery of targeted social change programs that are effective, efficient, and sustainable. However, substantial differences exist within the environment in which social marketing operates and the issues which form the basis of social campaigns. It is, therefore, not feasible to import commercial marketing practice wholesale into social marketing. Social marketing is the adaptation, rather than the direct transfer of marketing tools and techniques for social change campaigns.

Kotler and Lee (2008) defined social marketing as the use of marketing principles and techniques to create, communicate, and deliver value to the target audience, in order to change their behavior for the good of society as well as the target audience. Most social marketing activity is undertaken or funded by government agencies. While social marketing is an important part of government marketing, not all government marketing is social marketing, and not all social marketing activities are undertaken by the government. Social marketing is, however, a critical tool for effecting behavior change.

Social marketing is a part of the overall field of strategic marketing management, and it aims to achieve a voluntary behavior change based on providing a superior alternative to the present behavior. It does not coerce individuals into adapting or changing their behavior. Instead, the new behavior is "sold" to a target audience as a better lifestyle to adopt. Social marketing is, therefore, based on persuasion and not coercion. Based on the focus on individual voluntary behavioral change, social marketing is a customer-driven activity. Smoking and drinking reduce health, while exercise and vitamin consumption improves health. The world over, social marketing campaigns have been run to encourage people to abstain from risky sexual behaviors, smoking, alcohol abuse, and other health-endangering behaviors.

Social marketing is attracting the interest of both for-profit and not-for-profit institutions for the marketing of their services. Social marketing has a wider scope, and its techniques have been used successfully in promotional programs such as family welfare, heart care, physical fitness, immunization, awareness against HIV/AIDS, smoking, and drinking. Social marketing techniques are also being applied in important areas such as the provision of safe drinking water, soil and environmental conservation, forestation, and so on. Social leaders have been applying social marketing strategies in areas like the protection of human rights, the abolition of female genital mutilation, child labor, and domestic abuse.

Government institutions have been applying social marketing techniques in the implementation of their policies to ensure the long-term welfare of the society, especially in the face of the marketing of consumer products that prove dangerous to society and the environment. Imbalanced ecology has endangered the lives of people across the world, and yet is promoted by products used in daily life. For example, some detergents used for clothes washing are responsible for water pollution and loss of aquatic beings. Popular plastic products that are not properly disposed of will also create environmental problems. Additionally, many vehicles add to air and sound pollution. Several research studies have shown that consumables, like tobacco and alcoholic products, as well as cosmetics, are injurious to the health of its consumers. Notwithstanding government efforts to control the sale of such products, there are still dangerous products being poured into the market every day by businesses that seek to amass shareholder value against the public interest. These indifferent attitudes of such enterprises, as well as some marketers, have wrought irreparable damage to human life and the environment. Their application of wrong marketing strategies such as lying, omitting the truth, and false advertising has resulted in creating health problems, pollution, and ecological imbalance, the cost of which must be borne by the governments in most countries. The issues raised above make the adoption of social marketing practices very important to help educate the public so that they can adopt attitudes that will cause businesses not to harm the environment with their activities.

Government policy and strategy are progressively being reframed to focus more closely on the fundamental needs and concerns of individuals. Alongside this, the concentration at the local level is on guaranteeing the use of truly practical and steady approaches that can help people adopt and sustain an active and sound lifestyle. Social marketing is the tool that public agencies and NGOs utilize to facilitate behavioral change in target audience, through comprehensive and multifaceted approaches.

Social marketing as a discipline was "born" in the 1970s, when Kotler and Zaltman realized that the marketing principles that were applied in the sale of products to target audiences could be used to "sell" the idea of attitudinal and behavioral change. Since its distinction, social marketing has made enormous strides and has had a profoundly positive effect on social issues in the areas of general wellbeing, public health and safety, community involvement, and financial well-being. Kotler and Zaltman (1971) in defining social marketing, described it as the use of marketing principles to influence the acceptability of social ideas. Social marketing from their definition thus seeks to influence social behaviors that are beneficial to the general society and the target audience and not just the marketer. Social marketing draws from several bodies of knowledge, including psychology, sociology, political science, and communication theories with practical roots in advertising, public relations, and market research. It applies the principles and techniques drawn from commercial marketing to create awareness, encourage healthy behavior, and induce positive behavioral change in the target audience, thereby, improving the social, economic, and physical welfare of the individuals, organizations, or society as a whole. The underlying intent is to create positive social change.

There is difficulty in defining social marketing. For instance, scholars such as Rangun and Karim (1991), mention that Kotler and Zaltman's (1971) definition of social marketing is problematic. It is believed that terminology is a source of confusion. This is, because the terminology is often confused with societal marketing. The term social marketing comprises beliefs and changing attitudes. In most cases, the primary purpose is embarking on a campaign to influence behaviors for the good of the society. Another reason for the confusion of the terminology is whether social marketing practice is limited to public and nonprofit marketers. The debate was based on the fact that private organizations can also be involved themselves in social marketing. For instance, private firms like insurance companies can encourage drivers and passengers to use the seat belt while in a vehicle.

## Aspects of Social Marketing

Over the years, marketing practitioners and scholars have tried to identify essential features of social marketing. These can be summarized under need-based and eco-friendly product mix, rational promotional policy, reasonable price of the product, effective and efficient distribution, partnership between organizations and society, and suitable government policies.

### Need-Based and Eco-Friendly Product Mix

The social market product may be a physical product like contraceptives, services like health examinations, or ideas like environmental protection. The social marketer must make the people aware of their needs and problems and then sell the need-based products or services and not merely sell the products that the organization provides.

### Rational Promotional Policy

Social marketing sells ideas, thoughts, attitudes, and behaviors to promote social products. Social marketers use advertising media, public relations, door-to-door selling, and others to improve the acceptance of its products and services by the target audience. Social marketing gives emphasis on the adoption of the promotional policy by all organizations. Thus, the promotion of products/services should not be antisocial, anti-ethics, nor anti-ecology.

### Reasonable Price of the Product

The price of the social marketing product may be in the form of money, time, labor, or trouble. The social marketer has to adopt a reasonable pricing policy in which the benefits gained by the consumer are greater than the costs of the product. While making pricing decisions, the marketer must consider factors such as the purchasing power of the target groups and the quality of the product. Too high or too low prices of the products or service may get less or no response from the consumers.

### Effective and Efficient Distribution

Social marketing products may be tangible goods or intangible ideas, services, and practices. The social marketer has to provide social products to the customers at the right time and at the right place so that they are really benefited. The place of distribution should be well communicated and accessible to the consumers.

### Partnership Between Organizations and Society

Social marketing aims at achieving long term goals such as health promotion, production, population control, environmental conservation, and so on. These issues are complex and require combined efforts by various organizations to achieve better results.

### Suitable Government Policies

Social marketing programs may attract resistance from the target group. For example, the introduction of sex education at the school level may be opposed by some parents. Social marketing seeks political support to implement controversial social issues such as prevention of child marriages, encouraging birth control or family planning, educating the public on energy conservation, and so on. Many times, political diplomacy is needed to gain the support of the target group. While implementing social reform campaigns, the target group should be taken into consideration. This creates an environment suitable for the behavioral changes sought by social programs.

## The Public Sector Marketing Planning Process

A marketing plan is a blueprint or a written document that structures all of a firm's marketing activities, including the implementation and control of those activities. The influence of political figures is strongly felt in public services, especially by those public entities that receive funds only from the state budget. The decision-making power of these providers is limited since their responsibilities are limited to the management of state assets. Changes in government sometimes bring with them a change of national policy and strategies in accordance with the priorities established by the political leader during his or her candidacy in the bid to garner more votes.

Consequently, the objectives and initiatives of local public services providers can also be changed as they follow the established directives of the political leader. Real needs of citizens are therefore neglected and the public administration reform process is discontinuous, hence, the need for a strategic marketing plan in public service.

First, strategic marketing planning in the domain of public service must be the result of the cumulative efforts of different providers and institutions of the central government, especially ministries and institutions of local government administration. The stages of the corporate level planning in the public services field are the development of the government mission, naming the ministries, establishing the state budget, and allocating funds to various divisions. Thus, the main direction of a country is set by the government, which includes economic, cultural, and social policies. The government has the authority of the citizens to direct state institutions in order to achieve behavioral goals set out in the policies.

Public sector organizations adopt measures specific to the corporate or divisional level and strategic business units when they are planning their activities. They have the power in the management of public services and can choose one of the following forms of management: (direct, depersonalized, or autonomous administration), delegated (concession, lease, or interested administration), and half-direct (joint management). This is why a public institution, like any private firm, should "set up a specialized department and equip it to directly market and manage the institution's products and services and also deal exclusively with the review and revision process of their product portfolio" (Ionescu, 2011).

It can be noted that it is necessary to involve all stakeholders in the public sector in this highly complex and continuous process. Moreover, planning should not be carried out from top to bottom, but rather from the bottom-up. This means it should start from the functional levels of public service organizations and then go up to the corporate level where strategic decisions are adopted. To achieve this desideratum, public institutions should include their clients and other stakeholders in the planning process. This can provide useful information about the services they want, the quality or the accessibility thereof, and news about the services they may need in the future. Instruments of planning in the public enterprise are the mission, market segmentation, and positioning of the services in the minds of potential customers.

Secondly, all stakeholders involved in strategic marketing planning must have a common understanding of the institution's market position and image. Thus, there should be no inconsistencies between strategic and tactical decision-makers that unnecessarily complicate and prolong the process. In addition, the management of public enterprises should pay attention to the whole process of organizing work teams and training of their members. Planning teams will be composed of employees from several departments, so that all perspectives of constituent groups are known and coordinated by managers of functional areas within the organization. Following a general meeting, work teams will be informed and will receive instructions to begin and go through the above-mentioned process in order to set a high-quality level and determinants of this process, which are very important for any business.

Thirdly, the planning team must design some strategic options based on data collected from the market and a correct identification of an institution's competencies and weaknesses. Finally, the team must select the optimal strategy and develop the necessary plans.

## Conclusion

This chapter introduces the fundamentals and concepts of public sector marketing, recognizing how the government is deeply involved in healthcare provision in many ways. Unlike private healthcare with greater control over their marketing strategies, public sector providers take on a different marketing strategy. While private providers may not act in the public interest (e.g., a for-profit hospital that skimps on medical care because skimping is hard to detect), government provision may be superior to private sector provision. The chapter further explored the nuances of public sector marketing, focusing on the importance and challenges.

Marketing mix was presented as a necessary component to an organization's strategy for the completion of the objectives of the chapter moved beyond the actual 4Ps to introduce the 7Ps, which is also referred to as the expanded marketing mix. The elements within the marketing mix all affect the effectiveness of one another. A successful marketing mix will combine these variables in a way that will facilitate the attainment of organizational objectives.

The chapter further introduced different types of marketing in the public sector, with a greater focus on social marketing. The chapter concludes with the public sector marketing planning process, recognizing the influence of political figures on public healthcare provision, especially those healthcare providers who receive funds only from the state budget. The decision-making power of these providers is limited since their responsibilities are limited to the management of state assets. Changes in government sometimes bring with it a change of national policy and strategies following the priorities established by the political leader during his or her candidacy in the bid to garner more votes; hence, they need to have their strategic marketing plan in place to remain viable in the face of uncertainty.

## Review Questions

1. Define public sector marketing and explain how healthcare institutions in the public sector can adopt this concept?
2. Describe the marketing mix of public sector marketing with relevant examples.
3. Define social marketing and the different aspects as it relates to healthcare marketing.

---

### MINI-CASE: SOCIAL MARKETING — BREAST CANCER AWARENESS CAMPAIGN PROGRAM

In October 1997, a breast cancer awareness program (BRECAN) was launched in Nigeria to galvanize action against breast cancer as a life-threatening disease in Nigeria. BRECAN, a not-for-profit and nongovernmental organization, implemented the program through public sensitization, patient support, research, and advocacy.

Since 1997, BRECAN has sponsored several programs aimed at increasing breast health awareness and spurring action against all forms of cancer and breast cancer specifically. Some of the programs include the following:

1. *Jog for Life:* This home-grown, fun-filled outdoor event celebrates breast cancer survivors, increased awareness of the value of mammograms, raised funds to support research, and promoted exercise as a lifestyle. The lead jogger is usually an influencer woman in government (e.g., the state governor's wife).

2. *World Cancer Day:* This annual event is usually held on the 4th of February, a day chosen by the Union for International Cancer Control (UICC), a popular international cancer prevention organization in Switzerland. Nigeria's state Ministry of Health became a partner of BRECAN to mark the country's participation in World Cancer Day.
3. *Breast Cancer Awareness Outreach:* This outreach program targets women of all age groups, particularly women and young girls in secondary schools and higher institutions. The preventative value of breast self-examination is a feature of this program.
4. *Hope Lodge at BRECAN Center:* This center, established in 2010, offers lodging to breast cancer outpatients who are undergoing treatment at a university teaching hospital. BRECAN does this to ease accommodation challenges faced particularly by individuals who are indigent or who are unable to find housing for themselves or their families.
5. *Wellness Club:* As part of its effort to promote breast health education and cancer prevention through a healthy lifestyle, BRECAN's wellness club sponsors monthly breakfast aerobics programs. The Wellness Club was established in January 2012 and has become a popular attraction for women to support wellness through exercise.

Thus far, BRECAN has shown that a helping hand, no matter how small, can be a positive influence in the lives of cancer patients and their families. Some indigent patients receive financial assistance from funds generated internally even though it is not within the scope of the association to sponsor patient treatments. BRECAN's collaboration with a volunteer team of consultants at federal hospitals supports efforts to give women free access to clinical breast examinations. BRECAN believes that these actions and many more initiatives will alleviate breast cancer as a life-threatening disease in Nigeria.

This mini-case was developed by the authors using publicly available data.
Source: Breast Cancer Association of Nigeria (BRECAN). Available online at:
    http://brecan.org/about/

## Discussion Questions

1. How have the BRECAN programs had both short-term and long-term effects on breast cancer patients and survivors?

2. Describe three ways government agencies and other stakeholders (NGOs, the media, schools, and others) can assist BRECAN in achieving its aim of preventing or curing breast cancer?
3. BRECAN believes that its work will reduce the prevalence of breast cancer as a life-threatening disease and improve the lives of people touched by the ailment in Nigeria. Do you think this objective is achievable? What other steps can BRECAN take to achieve their objectives?

# References

Andreasen, A. R. (1994). Social marketing: Its definition and domain. *Journal of Public Policy and Marketing, 13*(1), 108–114.

Bagozzi, R. P. (1975). Marketing as exchange. *The Journal of Marketing, 39*(4,) 32–39.

Bang, H. P. (2003). New challenges to governance theory. In R. Mayntz (Ed.), *Governance as social and political communication* (pp. 27–40). Manchester, England: Manchester University Press.

Bauer, R. A. (Ed.). (1966). *Social indicators.* Oxford, England: Massachusetts Institute of Technology.

Bitner, M. J., & Booms, B. H. (1981). Trends in travel and tourism marketing: The changing structure of distribution channels. *Journal of Travel Research, 20*(4), 39–44.

Bouzas-Lorenzo, R. (2010). Public sector marketing, political science and the science of public administration: The evolution of a transdisciplinary dialogue. *International Review on Public and Nonprofit Marketing, 7*(2), 113–125.

Braveman, P. A., Kumanyika, S., Fielding, J., LaVesit, T., Borell, L. N., Manderscheid, R., & Troutman, A. (2011). Health disparities and health equity: The issue is justice. *American Journal of Public Health, 101*(S1), S149–S155.

Bruce, I. W. (1998). *Successful charity marketing: Meeting need.* Prentice Hall, Europe: ICSA.

Butler, P., & Collins, N. (1995). Marketing public sector services: Concepts and characteristics. *Journal of Marketing Management, 11*(1–3), 83–96.

Caruana, A. (2003). The impact of switching costs on customer loyalty: A study among corporate customers of mobile telephony. *Journal of Targeting, Measurement and Analysis for Marketing, 12*(3), 256–268.

Caruana, A., & Calleya, P. (1998). The effect of internal marketing on organizational commitment among retail bank managers. *International Journal of bank marketing, 16*(3), 108–116.

Caruana, A., Ramaseshan, B., & Ewing, M. T. (1997). Market orientation and organizational commitment in the Australian public sector. *International Journal of Public Sector Management, 10*(4), 294–303.

Cervera, A., Mollá, A., & Sanchez, M. (2001). Antecedents and consequences of market orientation in public organizations. *European Journal of Marketing, 35*(11/12), 1259–1288.

Day, G. S. (1998). What does it mean to be market-driven? *Business Strategy Review, 9*(1), 1–14.

Einbinder, L. C., & Schulman, K. A. (2000). The effect of race on the referral process for invasive cardiac procedures. *Medical Care Research and Review, 57*(S1), 162–180.

Ewing, M. T., & Caruana, A. (1999). An internal marketing approach to public sector management: The marketing and human resources interface. *International Journal of Public Sector Management, 12*(1), 17–29.

French, J., & Blair-Stevens, C. (2006). *Social marketing national benchmark criteria.* London, England: UK National Social Marketing Centre.

Gattinger, M. (2005). *A national energy strategy for Canada: Golden age or golden cage of energy federalism?: Canada: The State of the Federation, 2012. Regions, Resources, and Resiliency* (Working paper SOTF 2-12-04). Ontario, Canada: Institute of Governmental Relations.

Gelders, D., & Ihlen, O. (2010). Minding the gap: Applying a service marketing model into government policy communications. *Government Information Quarterly, 27*(1), 34–40.

Graham, P. (1994) Marketing in the public sector: Inappropriate or merely difficult?, *Journal of Marketing Management, 10*(5), 361–75.

Grigorescu, A. (2006). Marketing of public and private affairs–a link. *Kybernetes, 35*(7/8), 1179–1189.

Ionescu, F. T. (2011). Boston Consulting Group II–a business portfolio analysis matrix. *International Journal of Economic Practices and Theories, 1*(2), 65–70.

Kotler, P. (1982). *Marketing for nonprofit organizations.* Englewood Cliffs, NJ: Prentice-Hall.

Kotler, P., & Lee, N. (2008). *Corporate social responsibility: Doing the most good for your company and your cause.* Hoboken, NJ: Wiley.

Kotler, P., & Levy, S. J. (1969). Broadening the concept of marketing. *The Journal of Marketing, 33*(1), 10–15.

Kotler, P., & Zaltman, G. (1971). Social marketing: An approach to planned social change. *The Journal of Marketing, 35*(3), 8–12.

Laing, A. (2003). Marketing in the public sector: Towards a typology of public services. *Marketing Theory, 3*(4), 427–445.

Laing, A. W., & McKee, L. (2001) 'Willing volunteers or unwilling conscripts? Professionals and marketing in service organizations.' *Journal of Marketing Management, 17*(5–6), 559–576.

Lamb, C. W., Jr. (1987). Public sector marketing is different. *Business Horizons, 30*(4), 56–60.

Lazer, W., & Kelley, E. J. (1973). *Social marketing: Perspectives and viewpoints.* New York, NY: McGraw-Hill.

Lovelock, C. H., & Weinberg, C. B. (1990). *Public & nonprofit marketing: Readings and cases: Teaching notes.* San Francisco, CA: Scientific Press.

Mayntz, R. (2006). *The architecture of multi-level governance of economic sectors.* Köln, Germany: Max-Planck-Institut für Gesellschaftsforschung.

McCarthy, J. (1960). Recursive functions of symbolic expressions and their computation by machine, Part I. *Communications of the ACM, 3*(4), 184–195.

Peattie, S. (2003). Applying sales promotion competitions to nonprofit contexts. *International Journal of Nonprofit and Voluntary Sector Marketing, 8*(4), 349–362.

Peters, B. G., & Pierre, J. (1998). Governance without government? Rethinking public administration. *Journal of Public Administration Research and Theory, 8*(2), 223–243.

Rangun, V. K., & Karim, S. (1991). Teaching note: Focusing the concept of social marketing. Cambridge, MA: Harvard Business School.

Scrivens, E. (1991). Is there a role for marketing in the public sector? *Public Money and Management, 11*(2), 17–23.

Shapiro, B. P. (1973). Marketing for nonprofit organizations. *Harvard Business Review, 51*(5), 123–132.

Sheaff, R. (1991). *Marketing for health services: A framework for communications, evaluation, and total quality management.* Milton Keynes, England: Open University Press.

Sohn H. (2017). Racial and ethnic disparities in health insurance coverage: Dynamics of gaining and losing coverage over the life-course. *Population Research and Policy Review, 36*(2), 181–201.

Vigoda-Gadot, E., Shoham, A., Schwabsky, N., & Ruvio, A. (2005). Public sector innovation for the managerial and the post-managerial era: Promises and realities in a globalizing public administration. *International Public Management Journal, 8*(1), 57–81.

Walsh, K. (1991). Citizens and consumers: Marketing and public sector management. *Public Money and Management, 11*(2), 9–16.

Walsh, K. (1994). Marketing and public sector management. *European Journal of Marketing, 28*(3), 63–71.

Weinreich, D. M. (2003). Service-learning at the edge of chaos. *Educational Gerontology, 29*(3), 181–195.

Wilkinson, R. G. (1996). *Unhealthy societies: The afflictions of inequality.* London, England: Routledge.

Xia, L., & Monroe, K. B. (2004). Price partitioning on the internet. *Journal of Interactive Marketing, 18*(4), 63–73.

Zeithaml, V. A. (1988). Consumer perceptions of price, quality, and value: A means-end model and synthesis of evidence. *The Journal of Marketing, 52*(3), 2–22.

Zeithaml, V. A., Parasuraman, A., & Berry, L. L. (1985). Problems and strategies in service marketing. *Journal of Marketing, 49*(2), 33–46.

# 5

## Strategic Planning in Healthcare Marketing

### Chapter Outline

- Introduction
- Formulation of Vision, Mission, and Values
- Identifying Strategic Goals
- Strategic Analysis
- Strategy Formulation
- Strategy Implementation
- Strategy Evaluation
- Conclusion
- Review Questions
- Mini Case Study With Discussion Questions
- References

*Marketing in Healthcare-Related Industries*, pages 105–131
Copyright © 2020 by Information Age Publishing
All rights of reproduction in any form reserved.

## Chapter Outcome

By the end of this chapter, the reader will be able to

- understand how to formulate a strategy,
- understand the strategic planning process, and
- understand how to implement a strategy to achieve marketing goals.

## Introduction

The saying, "A healthy nation is a wealthy nation," represents the notion that a society's health and well-being is a necessity for the development of any nation. This is because most people need medical care at some point in their lifetime; since illnesses, accidents, and emergencies may arise, and there would be the need for hospitals and healthcare professionals to diagnose, treat, and manage them. Therefore, healthcare systems play an important role in the quality of life and social welfare of the people in the society. However, to have effective health systems that deliver value to patients, there is a need for strategic planning at every level of a nation's health delivery system. This chapter of the book treats strategic planning in healthcare. The chapter opens with an introduction to strategic planning and follows with the identification of strategic goals. It then addresses strategic analysis and strategy formulation. Strategy implementation is treated next to help readers understand how they can implement strategies that they formulate, and the chapter closes with the strategy evaluation.

## Strategic Planning

Strategic planning is the process that describes the direction a healthcare organization will pursue within its chosen environment in order to respond to the opportunities and challenges of the marketplace. For example, a healthcare organization may decide to serve the National Health Insurance Scheme (NHIS) cardholders to increase their clientele. Strategic planning guides the allocation of resources and efforts of the healthcare organization. According to Bryson (1988), strategic planning is fast becoming a part of the list of items to be attended to by a public planner. This suggests that strategic planning is not an activity that is restricted to for-profit health institutions alone, but it is useful for public sector health institutions as well. Berry (1994) suggests that strategic planning stakeholders in public institutions are demanding improved service and an improved sense of responsibility (Poister, Edwards,

Pasha, & Edwards, 2013) towards them. For public sector healthcare institutions, prominent advances in science and technology, as well as several facets of the financial, social, political, and economic life, have led to the growth and expansion of strategic planning throughout public administration (Bryson, 2011). Public sector health institutions have to be flexible; offer high-quality, valuable services; and move beyond just satisfying customers to please them. They should also welcome contributions from stakeholders and encourage employee buy-ins in order to stay relevant (Osborne & Gaebler, 1993) in an increasingly technological age. The world is fast becoming a global village and as such is a highly connected habitation (Orr, 2015), where the slightest change in one place has the possibility to echo unpredictably in other parts of the world (Bryson, 1999). Therefore, as purported by Osborne and Gaebler (1993), the quest for innovative, receptive, effective, and cost-efficient growth should be a good enough incentive to push healthcare institutions towards strategic planning.

The focus of strategic planning in healthcare marketing is basically to foster good relationships with various customer audiences. This can be attributed to the fact that it is the customer that determines the value of a service. When a healthcare provider can deliver value to its customer base, he is able to differentiate himself from competitors. Since healthcare is a dynamic industry and constantly changing, mainly due to changes in government policy, demographic structure, and technological and scientific advancements, strategic planning gives firms an imperative advantage, especially in a time of rapid advancements in technology as well as the regulation of healthcare firms and their performance. What is more, strategic planning serves as a means through which a firm responds to changes in the external environment, provides a mechanism of periodically repositioning an organization in its external environment, and allows for organizations to respond to fresh opportunities and challenges. In strategic planning, all the functional areas like finance, human resources, operations, and marketing develop their own plans.

A strategy aids in launching an orientation and direction towards a goal (or set of outcomes) within a particular context. It directs a firm's decision-making process by identifying how and what. Further, it puts everyone within the firm on track to achieve a common goal. Similarly, strategic planning is seen as a step-by-step approach that guides a firm in decision-making with regards to the required efforts and developments, considering the circumstances and atmosphere in which the firm functions. Primarily, strategic planning assesses the external atmosphere of the firm, examines the firm itself, detects main subjects to tackle, and then formulates strategies to guide the organization's procedures.

In the private sector, healthcare institutions' strategic growth often begins with the construction of the mission statement. In doing this, management of these firms can give thoughtful consideration to the firm's needs, thereby protecting the firm's welfare and taking decisions for the firm's advantage. Despite the diverse approaches and concerns that various stakeholders may have within a private firm, these stakeholders will still consider the firm's benefit to be their collective objective. For example, a private health institution may decide not to render its services to holders of the national health insurance card if it believes offering its services to them may have a negative effect on its cash flows and, hence, its ability to pay staff and medical suppliers on time.

For public sector healthcare institutions, the firm's obligation is often predetermined to a great extent and is implicit in the actual rationale underpinning the organization's very existence and survival. Similarly, the main obligation for which the firm came into being may have been susceptible to varying political ideas and public demands or may have been distorted with time. Hence, with regards to the public sector, as the firm's mission echoes the public obligation, it is important to assess the macroenvironment where the firm functions may reveal the extent of its public responsibility and determine the scope of its public requirement, before the accurate mission of the organization can be defined (Wilkinson & Monkhouse, 1994).

To develop an effective strategic plan, an organization must first define its vision and mission. Second is the situation analysis where the organization conducts an internal and external assessment of the threats and opportunities to which the organization may be exposed and also assesses its own distinctive competencies. Thirdly, the organization must establish a set of objectives based on critical factors emanating from the second stage, which must be aligned with the mission. Next, is to determine what marketing strategy should be deployed to achieve the identified objectives and to win in the marketplace.

### Vision

Unlike a mission, a vision statement is qualitative in nature. A vision statement is a declaration of a preferred future for the firm and not a statement of the purpose of the firm. A vision statement answers the question, "What do we hope to become?" (DuFour & Eaker, 1998). A vision is the ultimate goal of a firm's work and defines what it intends to accomplish with regards to "the better world" it is working towards. The question of whether a vision is attainable is crucial, and discussions concerning this question should be welcomed.

Comprehending the influence of vision is significant in setting the requisite amount of dynamic tension in the organization—too much, and it will not be credible, too little and it will not be motivating. Vision is also for stakeholder support—it is the basis for "buy-in."

According to Rüegg-Stürm and Gomez (1994), vision is found amid reality and perfection. There is a slight difference between a real vision that defines something likely to materialize in the future and an imaginary vision that is not likely to materialize. Furthermore, a robust vision is one that is shared by all. This implies that top management must ensure that the formulated vision is one that the workers in the organization have confidence in which they are prepared to adhere. The vision of the Department of Health in South Africa, for example, is a long and healthy life for all South Africans and this translated into a mission that reads "to improve health status through the prevention of illnesses and the promotion of healthy lifestyles and to consistently improve the healthcare delivery system by focusing on access, equity, efficiency, quality and sustainability." The vision statement of Mayo Clinic, "Mayo Clinic will provide an unparalleled experience as the most trusted partner for health care," signifies their hope of being the most trusted healthcare clinic and leader in clinical education and research.

### Mission

An organizational mission refers to its purpose of existence, defining who the organization is, its values, and the customers it wishes to service. The assessment of a healthcare organization's external environment in which it functions lays the foundation for the formulation of an appropriate mission statement. For instance, the mission of Ghana Health Service is to add to socioeconomic improvement by advancing healthcare through access to quality health for all individuals living in Ghana, by utilizing a very much inspired workforce. With this mission, the analysis of the external environment may unearth several modern prospects and constitutional responsibilities for the agency, for example, a 24-hour emergency response. This kind of assessment will identify the extent of the choices accessible in defining the mission of the healthcare agency of a government. This may involve considering either joining forces with other organizations in the creation of an all-inclusive social package or to offer the requisite services entirely self-sufficiently.

Even though in literature there exists no agreed-upon interpretation of a mission statement, several authors agree that mission statements are the initial phases in strategy formulation (Strong, 1997). Furthermore, businesses are perceived not to survive in the absence of a distinct mission statement and in fact, are predicted to fail according to most academics (Analoui & Karami, 2002). A successful mission statement must recognize the purpose of the business and what the customer wants. Mission statements should "set the tone for the organization and provide the management with a purposely broad set of directions for how it should develop further business strategies." (Berkowitz, 2016, p. 48). Thus, a good mission statement should state what the firm is (i.e., its purposes and goals) and embrace the expectations of a target audience. The mission statement of the Wits University Donald Gordon Medical Center (WDGMC) is "providing world-class medical academic training in South Africa." This is drawn from a vision to "train and retain highly skilled medical experts in South Africa, whilst also providing highly specialized patient treatment and care."

The missions of an organization can be either broad or narrow. What matters most is the development of a mission that has the greatest possibility to succeed in the competitive business environment.

In 2012, Eric Berkowitz argued in his *Essentials of Health Care Marketing* book that an effective mission statement should have the following constituents:

1. the basic good or service, prime market, and technology to be adopted in delivering the good or service;
2. organizational goals, such as growth, profitability, stability, or survival, strategically stated;
3. organizational philosophy—the code of behavior that guides the organization's operation;
4. organizational self-concept—a self-evaluation based on a realistic determination of its strengths and weaknesses; and
5. public image—how those outside the organization view the particular entity.

In addition, through an organization's mission statement, the organizational values should be communicated to employees in a manner that inspires them to commit and identify with the organization. The mission statement and values for the Onslow Memorial Hospital in Jacksonville, North Carolina is shown in Figure 5.1.

A mission statement that is interactive in nature, according to Nohria and Eccles (1992), should mobilize action through the creative use of language to appeal to the personal and collective identities of individuals. An explicit and authoritative statement of mission makes it possible for employees to make the connection between their values and the collective

**Onslow Memorial Hospital**

**Our Mission—What drives us**
The mission of Onslow Memorial Hospital is to provide excellent patient health services in a family centered-environment.

**Our Culture—What we are all about**
At Onslow Memorial Hospital, the clinical staff, non-clinical staff, healthcare providers and volunteers partner together with patients and their families to support the patient experience. We thrive on a shared passion to sense the needs of others through a patient- and family-centered care philosophy. We are driven by a set of core values to serve our community through human touch.

**Patient- and Family-Centered Care**
In our daily work, we support the following patient- and family-centered care principles: Dignity and respect, collaboration, participation, and information sharing. As a partner with the Institute for Patient- and Family-Centered Care since 2009, we have seen our culture flourish by collaborating with the patient and family, seeing them as essential members of the healthcare team.

**Hardwiring Excellence**
We have partnered with the Studer Group to support our journey toward excellence. Through this partnership we continue to learn and hardwire evidence-based best practices to improve the experience for our patients, families, staff members, and providers. It really is about getting back to the basics, engaging our passion to serve others, and committing to service and operational excellence.

You and your family are our purpose. You make our work worthwhile. You give us the opportunity to make a difference.

**We are Onslow; We are PROUD**
We want to ensure that the patient experience is not just positive, but ALWAYS positive. This is why our staff developed expected service behaviors. We are PROUD to be a member of the Onslow Team and PROUD to serve our community!

P—Positive First Impression

R—Responsive

O—Ownership

U—Unity

D—Demonstrates Compassion

**Figure 5.1**  Mission statement and values for the Onslow Memorial Hospital in Jacksonville, North Carolina. *Source:* https://www.onslow.org/organizational-values

values of the agency. These connections may be motivating on several counts, by increasing the likelihood that people will engage deeply in work, by incorporating the agency and its goals into the employee's sense of identity, and by making performance at work a significant component of the self-concept. These mechanisms improve performance by increasing the motivation of individual employees to work as a team and strive to achieve the mission of the institution (Weiss, 1996).

―――

### *Value Statements*

There exist divergent views among scholars and public servants with regard to the interpretation of the notion of values and the associated notions of principles and ethics. Values are elucidated here as systematic views that impact the selection we make among existing ways (Rokeach, 1973). The terms *values* and *ethics* are usually used interchangeably; however, they are different. Not all values are ethical values, that is, enduring beliefs as to right and wrong behavior. "Values can be ethical, unethical, or simply non-ethical" (Henry, 1998). Basically, ethical values are progressively seen as a subset of values (Kernaghan, 1994). "How must we behave in order to make our vision reality?" is one question that core value statements seek to answer (DuFour & Eaker; 1998).

In describing their work with business organizations, Blanchard, O'Connor, and Ballard (1997) argued, "When aligned around shared values and united in a common purpose, ordinary people accomplish extraordinary results and give their organization a competitive edge." Although their work and research were conducted in a profit-driven context, key concepts may arguably be applied to nonprofit organizations as well. Blanchard and O'Connor wrote of the importance for contemporary organizations to adopt key values such as honesty, fairness, and integrity in order to survive in the current economy.

Blanchard et al. (1997) further contend that organizations centered on powerful shared values report better service to their clientele, achieve higher profits, and a higher quality of working environments for their employees. The authors state that it is these shared values that act as the primary authority within an organization. Thus, values are the authority that all organizational members answer to in order for statements of organizational values or belief statements to be effective and meaningful to public organizations. They must be translated from esoteric statements of stakeholder beliefs into clear and concise statements of observable behaviors. In other words, statements of core values do not merely answer the question, "What do we believe?" but also address the question: "Based on our core beliefs, how will we behave within our organization in order to achieve our vision?"

The Mayo Clinic has one of the most comprehensive sets of value statements (see Figure 5.2). These value statements are put forward by the Mayo

**Mayo Clinic**

**Value Statements**
These values, which guide Mayo Clinic's mission to this day, are an expression of the vision and intent of our founders, the original Mayo physicians and the Sisters of Saint Francis.

**Respect**
Treat everyone in our diverse community, including patients, their families, and colleagues, with dignity.

**Integrity**
Adhere to the highest standards of professionalism, ethics, and personal responsibility, worthy of the trust our patients place on us.

**Compassion**
Provide the best care, treating patients and family members with sensitivity and empathy.

**Healing**
Inspire hope and nurture the well-being of the whole person, respecting physical, emotional, and spiritual needs.

**Teamwork**
Value the contributions of all, blending the skills of individual staff members in unsurpassed collaboration.

**Innovation**
Infuse and energize the organization, enhancing the lives of those we serve, through the creative ideas and unique talents of each employee.

**Excellence**
Deliver the best outcomes and highest quality service through the dedicated effort of every team member.

**Stewardship**
Sustain and reinvest in our mission and extended communities by wisely managing our human, natural, and material resources.

**Figure 5.2**   Mayo Clinic's value statements. *Source:* https://www.mayoclinic.org/about-mayo-clinic/mission-values

Clinic together with their mission statement which reads, "To inspire hope and contribute to health and well-being by providing the best care to every patient through integrated clinical practice, education and research."

## Strategic Goals and Objectives

Even though vision and mission statements are usually brief statements, they should be comprehensive, broad, all-encompassing, and far-reaching.

They can often seem overpowering and somewhat impossible to accomplish. The message behind sayings such as, "How do you eat an elephant? One bite at a time" and "A journey of a thousand miles begins with the first step," can suitably be applied in attaining a mission and vision (Grusenmeyer, 2009, p. 5). By creating goals and objectives, organizations can craft the "bites," the road map, and manageable stepping stones to achieve the mission, make the vision materialize, and steer the organization towards its intended path.

Goals are the big topics and ambiguous concepts, and objectives are the specific, measurable, attainable, relevant, and timed (SMART) stages through which goals are attained. As long as there are objectives, goals can be achieved. If organizations remember to "start small and break goals down to minuscule" with regards to identifying the guiding phases, they will be able to move in the desired direction. Realistically, just a number of people make errors in being overly detailed when it comes to goals and objectives, even though there is the likelihood that people may get stuck in providing details when stating goals and objectives.

Goals and objectives that are not detailed enough result in chaos and confusion on the part of those working to achieve them. Goals and objectives that are written down and well communicated tend to be very effective. Goals have no conviction and stay as mere ideas when not written down and as a result, cannot be accounted for. Written goals and objectives provide motivation and serve as a constant reminder to everyone on the way forward. Among the most essential attributes of a well-written objective are measurable results and a timeframe for completion. It is important to estimate results and evaluate the time it would take to accomplish set goals and objectives. This allows owners or managers to assess the achievement and progress of the entire business, as well as individuals and teams within the business. Having clearly defined/articulated goals and objectives also helps to maintain focus and a perspective, establishes priorities that lead to greater job satisfaction, and improves employee performance.

It is of great importance that healthcare institutions reevaluate and establish fresh goals and objectives when old ones are achieved since conditions are bound to change. Employees become bored, and business may come to a standstill if the healthcare firm fails to periodically set new or more challenging goals. Finally, to maintain enthusiasm and continued progress, healthcare managers must offer positive feedback and reward employees when goals are met.

## Strategic Analysis

Strategic analysis involves settling on subjective decisions that rely on information. Strategic analysis seeks to decide alternative strategies that could best empower the firm to accomplish its primary goals. The healthcare company's present systems, targets, and missions, combined with the external and internal audit information gives a premise for producing and assessing feasible alternative strategies. Unless a desperate situation confronts the healthcare firm that would cause a paradigm shift, alternative strategies should represent incremental steps that move the healthcare firm from its present position to a desired future position. Alternative strategies should not be random and disparate but should be pulled from the healthcare organization's goals' internal audit, external audit, vision, and mission.

### The Nature of Strategic Analysis

Strategic analysis can be described as "a theoretically informed understanding of the environment in which an organization is operating, together with an understanding of the organization's interaction with its environment in order to improve organizational efficiency and effectiveness by increasing the organization's capacity to deploy and redeploy its resources intelligently" (Worrall, 1998, p. 3). Although the description of the term may differ from scholar to scholar, the essential attributes commonly associated with strategic analysis are identification and evaluation of data relevant to strategy formulation and the classification of the external and internal environment to be analyzed.

When deciding on a strategy to execute, the healthcare strategist must create a manageable set of the most attractive alternative strategies from which to choose. The points of interest, impediments, expenses, and advantages of these techniques ought to be determined and examined during the decision-making process. Recognizing and assessing alternative strategies should also include a significant number of supervisors and workers, who have a deep understanding of the organization's vision and mission statements, have performed the external audit, and have conducted the internal audit. Agents from every office and division of the organization should be incorporated into the process to allow for organization-wide contributions and holistic deliberations. Workers involved in the strategic analysis are privy to the firms internal and external audit information. The company's mission statement, together with this information will assist employees in making sound decisions regarding those strategies that they think would be of most benefits to the organization. Creativity should be encouraged in this thought process. Successions of meetings should be held to deliberate and reflect on the alternative strategies suggested. Suggested strategies should be written. After all the possible strategies have been identified, the strategies should be graded based on an appeal by all members. The end result of this is that the best strategies will be prioritized, and it will represent the collective insight of all members.

## Methods of Strategic Analysis of the Internal Healthcare Environment

The following are methods of stategic analysis which can be applied to the internal healthcare environment. These include the method "Tree of Aims," LOTS method and MOST model (Rudnicki, & Vagner, 2014).

### The Method "Tree of Aims"

This approach shows the codification of a pyramid of goals that highlights their differences and how they are interrelated. It is a graphic chart that shows how broader goals are translated into more specific goals. The topmost part of the chart indicates a dome between the goals. The strategy "tree of aims" is a key general approach for framework inquiry.

### LOTS Method

This method involves a thorough step-by-step dialogue on the numerous business concerns at different phases and diverse extents of complexities. This also includes the organization's main purpose and its current status, human resource, development plans, management reporting, and long- and short-term goals.

### MOST Model

Several models remove the hierarchy between the goals, techniques, and mission. The situation of a business entity is portrayed with indistinct criteria in relation to the MOST model. This may include an organization's installment of profits, overall revenues, and deals volume of various workers.

## Methods of Strategic Analysis of the External Healthcare Environment

The following are methods of stategic analysis which can be applied to the external healthcare environment (Rudnicki, & Vagner, 2014).

### The Ansoff Growth Matrix

This growth matrix by Ansoff is one of the approaches to marketing, which aids an organization in decision-making regarding its market growth strategy and products as well. This product/market matrix suggests that organizations attempt to expand their activities by either promoting novel or current products in prevailing or novel markets. The resultant effect of this product or market matrix is the development of outcome from the projected growth strategies, which sets the pace for the firm's technique.

### Porter's 5-Forces Model

Porter acknowledged five competitive forces from the influence of the business at the market and the level of benefits (Porter, 1985). These forces include the influence of suppliers, the impact of buyers' strength, existing competitors in the industry, the risk from the issue of substitute products, and new competitors who get into the industry and produce similar goods. Porter acknowledged three main techniques that can be linked to the competitive forces:

- Leadership strategy influences the firm to produce large amounts of goods in a big market.
- Strategy of product differentiation is applied in a case where the business with an exclusive access offer enters a deep market.
- Focus strategy emphasizes on limited geographic segments and one segment of the market.

### The BCG Strategic Portfolio Model

The Boston Consulting Group (BCG) strategic portfolio model was established by the Boston Consulting Group. It is a growth-share portfolio planning model used to strategically assess the status of an organization's brand portfolio. Fundamentally, the premise of this model is that a firm will have its expenditure reduced and revenue increased if that firm has a relatively high market share. The framework also categorizes firms pertaining to their growth and profit potential. Further, it involves the employment of numerical equations in estimating the growth and profit potential. Within the BCG growth matrix framework, every item is classified either as a star, dog, cash cow, or problem child.

Cash cows signify those that have a high market share in slow-growing industries. These product are produced at a relatively minimal cost and they normally yield excess revenue for the firm.

Dogs represent those product lines with a low market share in slow-growing industries that basically yield sufficient revenue to sustain their market share. These products usually break even.

In relation to products termed as a problem child, they are usually those product lines with low market share in a highly developed market. They are generally the starting point for most businesses and require huge investments to turn them to "stars."

Star product lines typically have a high market share in a fast-growing industry. They are the improved versions of "problem children" and possess the ability to become future "cash cows" if they are properly managed.

**GE McKinsey Matrix**

The GE McKinsey matrix is comparable to the BCG growth-share matrix, in that it plots the Strategic Business Unit (SBU's) position in the industry and plots the strategic business units on a grid of the industry. The GE matrix, however, is an expanded version of the BCG. The GE matrix generalizes the axes as *business unit* and *industry attractiveness* instead of *market growth* and *relative market share*. Also, the GE matrix has nine cells instead of the four cells in the BCG matrix.

The nine cells GE is preferable to the four cells BCG matrix because it offers a better graphic representation of a firm's position within the matrix. Further, unlike the BCG, where the *invest* and *harvest* cells are more together and may complicate decision-making, the GE McKinsey clearly shows the difference between those cells that are harvested and those that are invested in.

One other motive behind the existence of the GE McKinsey is that the guys at General Electric found the BCG less refined or sophisticated. In BCG, a firm's competitive advantage depends on its market share. Thus, a firm is better positioned in the market if its market share is relatively large. Even though this assumption holds water, market share is not the only determinant of competitive advantage. As such, this assumption tends to oversimplify the issue. In addition, with the BCG matrix, industry attractiveness has been used as the only determinant of market growth rate which is yet again another shortfall of the BCG matrix; no wonder a complicated business portfolio like General Electrics necessitated a more robust tool than the BCG.

**Thompson and Strickland Method**

This method predicts corporate-level decisions with a basis on two factors: competitive advantage (weak or strong) and market growth rate (slow or rapid). The potential strategic options are positioned in order to mini-mize their appeal within the matrix.

### 7S McKinsey Model

This approach is used to ascertain the key internal factors impacting an organization's current state and expected growth. The 7s model entails strategy, structure, systems, staff, style (management style), skills, and shared values (Waterman, Peters, & Philips, 1980). The foremost three attributes are usually considered manageable, more tangible, and quantifiable. They are commonly referred to as "hard." The remaining attributes are usually seen not to be easily controlled and as such, instead of management, lead-ership is required to put them in check; they are referred to as "soft."

### Arthur D. Little (ADL)/Life Cycle (LC) Matrix

The basis for this model is that, just as human beings, businesses also pass through growth phases (life cycles). The ADL model is a portfolio management approach that is grounded in the product life cycle philoso-phy. It employs the aspects of a firm's competitive advantage and that of environmental assessment. The ADL/LC matrix is typically applicable; its application is particularly suited to small firms and for Small Business Units (SBU) of big firms.

### Hofer/Schendel Model

This type of model is directed at how firms position themselves in the matrix of goods development and the establishment of an optimal set of business. Ordinarily, two ideal sets of business exist: selling the old business or acquiring a new one. Nonetheless, the conditions surrounding each one depends on the extent of productivity in relation to competitors and mar-ket development.

### PEST Analysis

PEST (political, economic, social, and technological analysis) is an ac-ronym for the four main factors in an organization's external environment. Fundamentally, it is a strategic planning tool that aids firms in ascertaining how these factors influence business activities. Other researchers often add demographics, ecology, and legislation, to the four factors mentioned above.

### SWOT Analysis

SWOT is an acronym for strength, weakness, opportunities and threats. SWOT analysis is among the most well-known approaches of strategic analysis which includes factors of both the internal and the external environment, making it possible to assess prevailing potential threats and opportunities of the firm, as well as to create a strategy for extra growth. For example, the introduction of the national health insurance policy offers healthcare institutions an opportunity to increase its market share, with the insurance policy making healthcare accessible to people who formally could not access healthcare due to the cost involved.

## Strategy Formulation

The process by which an organization selects the utmost suitable courses of action to attain its defined goals is known as strategy formulation. This process is vital to a firm's achievement because it offers a model for the actions that will result in the expected outcomes. Strategy formulation refers to the process of selecting the utmost suitable course of action for the recognition of the goals and aims of the organization and by so doing, will help achieve the vision of the organization. There are six main steps in the process of strategy formulation, which are detailed below.

### Setting Organizations' Objectives

The main element of any strategy statement is to set the long-term aims of the firm. It is recognized that strategy is commonly a medium for the realization of objectives of the organization. Objectives stress the state of "being there," whereas strategy stresses upon the process of "reaching there." Strategy contains both the addition of objectives and the means used to achieve those objectives. Therefore, strategy is a broader term which outlines the deployment of resources to attain the objectives.

### Evaluating the Organizational Environment

Evaluating the organizational environment is the next step after setting the organizational objectives. It encompasses a review of the competitive position of the organization which must start with a quantitative or qualitative review of the existing services offered by the healthcare institution. The reason for this review is to ensure that the factors essential for competitive success in the market can be uncovered in order for the management of the health institution to recognize their weaknesses and strengths as well as those of their competitors. After recognizing the strength and weaknesses of the healthcare institution, it is up to the institution's management to again monitor the "doings" or actions of their competitors. This will help the health institution to uncover the opportunities and threats in the business environment, its market, or supply sources.

### Setting Quantitative Targets

With the setting of quantitative targets, a healthcare institution can fix the quantitative target values for some of its objectives. By setting targets for new customers, a comparison can be made with the numbers of long-term customers in order to assess the contribution that might be made by the operating departments or numerous product and service zones.

### Aiming in Context With the Divisional Plans

When a healthcare institution aims in context with its divisional plans, contributions made by each division, service product category, or each department within the institution are recognized, and strategic planning is done for each subunit. This necessitates a careful examination of the trends in the macroeconomic environment.

### Performance Analysis

This includes uncovering and investigating the gap between the desired performance and the planned performance. A crucial assessment of the firm's past performance, current situations, and the desired future situations must be done by the firm. This crucial assessment recognizes the degree of gap that continues to exist between the actual reality and the long-term aspirations of the firm. An effort is made by the firm to estimate its possible future situations if the present trends persevere.

### Choice of Strategy

Choice of strategy is the final step in the formulation of the strategy. The best choice of strategy is selected after bearing in mind the goals of the organization, potential and limitations, and strengths, as well as the external opportunities.

## Strategy Implementation

Implementing strategy is often more difficult than formulating it, and as a result, it has become an aspect of management where many organizations fail. The actual value of a decision surfaces only after the decision is implemented. In other words, making a good decision is not enough to achieve effective results unless the decision is adequately implemented. Implementing strategy effectively involves working the entire organizational structure in a concerted effort to implement strategic initiatives, advance the strategic agenda, and move an organization into the future in a deliberate manner. Implementation refers to how a firm's plans are translated into actionable tasks and are shaped in a way that achieves the goals outlined in a company's plan. Implementation is a series of interventions related to organizational structures, key personnel actions, and control systems designed to monitor performance with respect to desired ends. Implementation designates the managerial interventions that align organizational action with strategic intention (Noble, 1999). Implementation can be described as the sum total of the activities and choices required for the execution of a strategic plan, and the process by which strategies and policies are put into action (Smith & Kofron, 1996).

Public agencies, including healthcare institution, can develop action plans for implementing a particular strategic initiative and utilize project management approaches to ensure that the strategy is carried out to completion. Strategy implementation is the communication, interpretation, adoption, and enactment of strategic plans, and it is widely perceived to be a significant determinant of performance. As stated by Long and Franklin (2004), when studying strategy implementation, a key variable is the approach that is used to implement it. In discussing the processes used to put strategy into practice, there is a range of possible implementation styles suggested by Bourgeois and Brodwin (1984), with rational implementation at one end of the spectrum and incremental implementation at the other. Implementation style is the approach organizations use when practicing strategies. Two main elements exist for this: the degree to which responsibility is centralized or decentralized and whether creation and execution are distinct and chronological activities or are entangled. An organization's implementation style forms part of its administrative routine, which is recognized as crucial to understanding the dynamics of implementation.

A rational implementation style is characterized by centralized control, the use of formal means to secure compliance, and the separation of formulation and implementation. Strategy formulation and implementation are, however, sequential. There can be no implementation of a strategy if it has not been previously deliberately formulated. As part of its evaluation of appropriate strategies, an organization is likely to pilot the strategy before full implementation (Bryson, 1995). Successful implementation of change is dependent on several factors; one of which is the drafting of a plan which will function as an organizational roadmap. Formal methods, such as business or project plans, which help clearly define activities by identifying tasks and targets, are likely to be used by rational implementers in the implementation process. Control has also been identified as central to the implementation process, and in rational approaches, this is done centrally through techniques such as action plans and monitoring.

Incremental implementation style decentralizes responsibility and has a much looser distinction between strategy formulation and implementation. It is argued that the separation of formulation and implementation, as given in the rational approach, is a key reason for implementation failure (Mintzberg, 1994). Organizations can learn more effectively and respond to changes in the environment by connecting these processes (Montgomery, 2008). In an incremental style, the responsibility for implementation is decentralized and the role of organizational members is enhanced as they take an active part in the process of developing and implementing the strategy.

In implementing strategy, organizations allocate special tasks and roles to the employees and state how these tasks and roles can be correlated to maximize efficiency, satisfy customers, and achieve competitive advantage. The following are the main steps in implementing a strategy:

- Develop an organization's potential for carrying out strategy effectively.
- Disburse abundant resources to strategy-essential activities.
- Create policies that encourage strategy.
- Employ the best policy programs and practices for constant improvement.
- Link reward structures to the accomplishment of results.
- Make use of strategic leadership.

Exceptionally formulated strategies will fail if they are not properly implemented. And as such, it is essential to note that strategy implementation is not possible unless there is a stability between strategy and each organizational element, such as organizational structure, reward structure, resource-allocation, and processes.

## Strategy Evaluation

Strategy evaluation is not an entirely new concept to public administration as evaluation is a regulatory requirement. Strategy evaluation is alleged to have begun in the 1930s in Sweden's public sector. It provides organizations with an accurate picture of what is happening regarding the implementation of the strategy. The purpose of strategy evaluation is to outline divergences and unravel all limitations within the strategy implementation process. It is unlikely to predict all the glitches that may emerge during strategy formulation. Therefore, both strategy formulation and strategy evaluation are of equal importance. Consequently, it is important that strategy implementation procedures are assessed by management in order to review and shape the strategy implementation approach.

During this phase (strategy evaluation) of the strategic management procedure, strategists attempt to offer surety that the organization's chosen strategy has been accurately executed and it is right on course in terms of the organizational goals. Strategists attempt to determine if the chosen strategy has resulted in any diversions of real performance. With this information, managers can then take appropriate actions to resolve issues and make the strategy unfold as planned. After this is done, curative measures are put in place to address these issues. In cases where there is a divergence, real-time feedback is crucial as this aids management to act in a timely manner. Hence, evaluation requires that an effective system is put in place to make this possible. In practice, strategy evaluation requires a system of controls. The system helps managers to monitor the progress of a strategic plan. Strategy evaluation and control systems help managers to find out the following:

- Are the firms' policies in line with the decisions being made by those implementing the strategy?
- Are sufficient resources being distributed and are they being judiciously used?
- Are the predicted events in the external atmosphere real?
- Are the long-term and short-term goals being met?
- Are the strategists on course?

Some of the reasons for the need to evaluate strategy are discussed next:

1. Organizations are constantly faced with dynamic environmental factors that change quickly. These changes affect strategy implementation, and the regular evaluation of strategy implemented, provides relevant data for taking corrective actions.
2. Installation of an evaluation system with well-stated timelines pushes authorities to frequently assess the impact of variations in the organizational environment and the implemented strategy. This keeps them in check and reminds them that there is always

room for improvement and that, whatever is accomplished in present times is not an assurance of future achievements.

Strategy evaluation consists of the following steps:

1. *Create benchmarks:* Benchmarks should be created to evaluate the effectiveness of strategy performance. To determine performance benchmarks, it is essential to discover the requirements for performing the task. Pointers that best describe the performance and express requirements of a task can be determined and used for evaluation when these benchmarks are set. Organizations can use both quantitative and qualitative criteria for a comprehensive assessment of performance. Quantitative criteria entail ascertaining net profit, rate of laborer, ROI, labor turnover, learning on shares, production cost, and rate of labor turnover. Qualitative factors are subjective evaluation and include factors such as risk-taking potential, skills and competencies, and flexibility.

2. *Measurement of performance:* Real performance is likened to the expected performance, which serves as the target. Performance is assessed with the aid of communication and reporting system. Strategy evaluation is less problematic if targets are accurately set and correct approaches are used in the assessment of performance. However, it will still be problematic to measure elements such as managers' inputs. Likewise, measuring a factor like divisional performance is mostly difficult; therefore, goals that are set must be adjustable alongside those aspects of performance that are quantifiable. If the assessment is not done at the appropriate time, the purpose for evaluation may be defeated.

3. *Analyzing variance:* In determining real performance by relating it to expected performance, differences may perhaps exist which the institution will have to examine. The degree of tolerance limits for the variance between expected and real performance should be outlined. A negative divergence reveals underperformance, and as such, curative procedures should be put in place to check the issue. On another hand, positive divergence indicates improved productivity even though it is uncommon to continually surpass the benchmark.

4. *Taking corrective action:* It is of pertinence to put in place curative measures after a deviation is detected in assessing actual performance. In a case where expected performance persistently exceeds real performance, a thorough examination of the reasons behind such performance is carried out. Further, strategists may consider dropping standards if they detect the prerequisites for

performance are not in line with the firm's potential. In addition, although an unusual curative procedure, strategists may also decide to recreate the strategy, which may demand to reformulate new strategies in distributing resources as well as a total restructuring of the strategic management procedures.

## Conclusion

For healthcare providers to remain viable, strategic planning is very important, putting plans in place to describe the direction in which the organization wants to go. Strategic planning is the process that describes the direction of a healthcare system. This includes documenting their values in the form of organization vision, mission, and strategic goals and objectives. Formulating these strategies can be daunting, but it is very important as the process is vital to a firm's achievement. It offers a model for the actions that will result in the expected outcomes. The six main steps in the process of strategy formulation were discussed.

The chapter also highlighted that implementing strategy is often more difficult than formulating it, and it is an aspect of management where many organizations fail. The organization should be able to translate the plans into actionable tasks and are shaped in a way that achieves the goals outlined in a company's plan. This includes working along with their staff and stakeholders to make sure these objectives are met.

Evaluating these strategies were also considered essential. Though the plan has been written and implemented, the organization needs to review how well the plan is being followed and the outcome—perhaps they may need to change goals they have achieved and set new goals. With this information, managers can then take appropriate actions to resolve issues and make the strategy unfold as planned. After this is done, curative measures are put in place to address these issues.

## Review Questions

1. Describe strategic planning.
2. Explain how organizations can formulate their strategic plans.
3. Explain the importance of strategic plan evaluation.

## MINI CASE STUDY: LAYING OUT THE BLUEPRINT

Mark Appiah received the call he had earnestly longed for: to accept the position as administrator of Hilltop Family Clinic (HFC) in Accra, Ghana. Mark would be the first professional administrator in the clinic's 10-year history. Hilltop Clinic was owned by Dr. Emmanuel Kwasi, a family medicine specialist. Though the clinic had experienced substantial growth, Dr. Kwasi desired more progress. He had observed some deficiencies in operations, which he attributed to lack of foresight and knowledge on the part of the administrator, Sarah Kofi. The doctor was committed to future expansion for his medical practice and felt that a well-planned marketing strategy would attract patient traffic, a result that would require the services of a doctor, a pediatrician, and a neurologist to add to his current staff of two general practitioners. Fortunately, Sarah was about to retire, thus, allowing for a smooth transition to professional management practices.

Mark began work at HFC on a Monday morning, which was Sarah's last official day as a clinic administrator. She gave him a thorough tour of the clinic, and he had a congenial meeting with Dr. Kwasi for several hours. On the second day of Mark's new job, he received a troubling letter from a patient, which was addressed to the office of the administrator. The letter read thus:

Kofi Benson
Accra, Ghana.
10th January 2017

The Administrator,
Hilltop Family Clinic,
Accra, Ghana

Dear Sir/Madam,

**LETTER OF COMPLAINT**

On Saturday the 5th day of January 2019, I received a call around 12:30 p.m. that my 71-year-old grandfather had experienced an eyeball rupture and was in severe pain. We immediately rushed him to your clinic for treatment since he is a registered patient of HFC. After waiting for two hours, the doctor told us he could not handle such an emergency and referred us to Divine-Grace General Hospital. The doctor promised to send my grandfather's medical history to Divine-Grace so the doctors there would attend to him without delay or further questioning, especially since it was clearly an emergency.

Your clinic called the ambulance service to take my grandfather to the hospital.

We arrived at Divine-Grace Hospital in the afternoon about 3:30 p.m., and to my amazement, my grandfather was required to undergo the patient registration process and would have to wait his turn to see the doctor before any treatment would be offered, and there were many people waiting to see the doctor. We had been assured by your clinic that my grandfather's medical history would be rushed to the Divine-Grace administrative office so there wouldn't be any need for admitting procedures or consultation, but their office assured me that they had not received any such report from your clinic. We had no choice but to get a card for him, open a case file, and join those at the waiting area.

My grandfather was in severe pain with blood oozing slowly out of his eyes. At about 6:00 p.m., I pleaded with one of the nurses to at least put some medication or bandages on his eye to give him some relief. We were given a gauze pad which we held to his face, and after another hour we were told we would have to leave because the hospital staff who could help him were leaving for the weekend and would return on Monday. My grandfather endured a painful weekend. We returned the following Monday at 4:00 a.m. so he could be first in line for treatment when the staff returned at 7:00 a.m. We were seen first, and he was able to receive treatment that immediately relieved his pain.

I am writing this letter to you because even when we returned to Divine-Grace Monday, my grandfather's medical records from your clinic had still not reached there. Given the communication technology available to medical practices today, it is highly disappointing that HFC failed in this regard despite its good quality of service. It should not have taken more than 10 minutes to forward my grandfather's report to Divine-Grace. I had expected that when we arrived at the hospital, my grandfather would be attended to immediately.

I hope this issue is looked into. HFC patients should expect that your clinic will keep pace with ongoing advancements in administrative techniques and procedures.

Yours faithfully,

Kofi Benson

After Mark had read the letter, it became clear to him that he had been hired to help create a professional healthcare delivery. He went to work documenting ongoing administrative and clinical practices, so he could submit a preliminary report to Dr. Kwasi that would clearly state his observations and plans for improved administrative practices. He was able to identify good practices that should be sustained as well as weaknesses that he was determined to abolish. Good practices included the delivery of quality healthcare services to patients and a serene physical environment. The glaring weakness corresponded with the issues raised in Kofi Benson's letter. HFC lacked advanced administrative techniques and procedures, and found these fundamental practices to be lacking:

1. detailed standard operating procedures to guide processes and practices,
2. a mission statement that would establish expectations,
3. detailed job description for each staff member,
4. code of conduct guiding behaviors at the workplace,
5. marketing efforts that would replace word-of-mouth referrals, and
6. management involvement and support.

Mark was determined to develop and implement a service blueprint that would allow for professional business practices in the hospital.

### Discussion Questions

1. Imagine you are a patient who visited the clinic and found the waiting room filled with both emergency and non-emergency cases. What do you think the clinic staff can do to help patients in this situation? What administrative efforts should Mark put in place to make Hilltop Family Clinic your healthcare provider of choice? What marketing activities can be put in place to support those efforts?
2. What should a typical standard operating procedure of a clinic include?

## References

Analoui, F., & Karami, A. (2002). CEOs and development of the meaningful mission statement. Corporate governance. *The International Journal of Business in Society, 2*(3), 13–20.

Berkowitz, E. N. (2016). *Essentials of health care marketing.* Burlington, MA: Jones & Bartlet.

Berry, S. T. (1994). Estimating discrete-choice models of product differentiation. *The RAND Journal of Economics, 25*(2), 242–262.

Blanchard, K. H., O'Connor, M. J., & Ballard, J. (1997). *Managing by values.* San Francisco, CA: Berrett-Koehler.

Bourgeois, L. J., & Brodwin, D. R. (1984). Strategic implementation: Five approaches to an elusive phenomenon. *Strategic Management Journal, 5*(3), 241–264.

Bryson, A. E. (1999). *Dynamic optimization.* New Jersey, NJ: Prentice Hall.

Bryson, J. (1988). Strategic planning: Big wins and small wins. *Public Money & Management, 8*(3), 11–15.

Bryson, J. M. (1995). *Strategic for public and nonprofit organizations: Guide to strengthening and sustaining organizational achievement.* San Francisco, CA: Jossey-Bass.

Bryson, J. M. (2011). *Strategic planning for public and non-profit Organizations: A guide to strengthening and sustaining organizational achievement.* San Francisco, CA: Jossey-Bass.

DuFour, R., & Eaker, R. (1998). *Professional learning communities at work: Best practices for enhancing student achievement.* Bloomington, IN: National Education Service.

Grusenmeyer, D. (2009). Mission, visions, values, & goals. Farm Business Study Unit. Cornell University, Ithaca, NY. Retrieved from https://ecommons.cornell.edu/bitstream/handle/1813/36906/pdmission.pdf?sequence=1&isAllowed=y

Henry, C. R. (1998). Surface studies of supported model catalysts. *Surface Science Reports, 31*(7–8), 231–325.

Kernaghan, K. (1994). The emerging public service culture: Values, ethics, and reforms. *Canadian Public Administration, 37*(4), 614–630.

Long, E., & Franklin, A. L. (2004). The paradox of implementing the government performance and results act: Top–down direction for bottom–up implementation. *Public Administration Review, 64*(3), 309–319.

Mintzberg, H. (1994). *The rise and fall of strategic planning.* New York, NY: Free Press.

Montgomery, M. R. (2008). The urban transformation of the developing world. *Science, 319*(5864), 761–764.

Noble, C. H. (1999). The eclectic roots of strategy implementation research. *Journal of Business Research, 45*(2), 119–134.

Nohria, N., & Eccles, R. G. (1992). *Networks and organizations.* Boston, MA: Harvard Business School Press.

Orr, R. C. (2015, April 18). *Making public policy in the 21st century.* Retrieved from http://publicpolicy.umd.edu/sites/default/files/UMD%20SPP%20The%20Policy%20E xchange%202015_01.pdf

Osborne, D., & Gaebler, T. (1993). Reinventing government: The five strategies for reinventing government. *Public Productivity and Management Review, 16*(4), 349–356.

Poister, T. H., Edwards, L. H., Pasha, O. Q., & Edwards, J. (2013). Strategy formulation and performance: Evidence from local public transit agencies. *Public Performance & Management Review, 36*(4), 585–615.

Porter, E. M. (1985). *Competitive advantage.* New York, NY: The Free Press/Macmillan.

Rokeach, M. (1973). *The nature of human values.* New York, NY: Free Press.

Rudnicki, W., & Vagner, I. (2014). Methods of strategic analysis and proposal method of measuring productivity of a company. *Zeszyty Naukowe Małopolskiej Wyższej Szkoły Ekonomicznej w Tarnowie, 25*(2), 175–184.

Rüegg-Stürm, J., & Gomez, P. (1994). From reality to vision—from vision to reality—an essay on vision as medium for fundamental knowledge transfer. *International Business Review, 3*(4), 369–394.

Smith, K. A., & Kofron, E. A. (1996). Toward a research agenda on top management teams and strategy implementation. *Irish Journal of Management, 17*(1), 135–152.

Strong, C. (1997). The problems of translating fair trade principles into consumer purchase behavior. *Marketing Intelligence & Planning, 15*(1), 32–37.

Waterman, R. H., Jr., Peters, T. J., & Phillips, J. R. (1980). Structure is not organization. *Business Horizons, 23*(3), 14–26.

Weiss, J. A. (1996) Public management and psychology. In D. Kettl & B. Milward (Eds.), *The state of public management* (pp. 118–143). Baltimore, MD: Johns Hopkins University Press.

Wilkinson, G., & Monkhouse, E. (1994). Strategic planning in public sector organizations. *Executive Development, 7*(6), 16–19.

Worrall, L. (1998). *Strategic analysis: A scientific art.* Wolverhampton, England: Wolverhampton Business School.

# 6

## *Managing Innovation in Healthcare Institutions*

### Chapter Outline

- Introduction
- Uncertainty in Healthcare Institutions
- Technical Uncertainty
- Market Uncertainty
- Managing Uncertainty in Healthcare Institutions
- Organizational Structure and Innovations
- Flexibility
- Communication
- Interorganizational Relationships
- Conclusion
- Review Questions
- Mini Case Study With Discussion Questions
- References

*Marketing in Healthcare-Related Industries,* pages 133–143
Copyright © 2020 by Information Age Publishing
All rights of reproduction in any form reserved.

**133**

## Chapter Outcome

By the end of this chapter, the reader will be able to

- describe uncertainty in healthcare institutions and its implication on marketing strategy,
- explain how innovations can be communicated in the context of healthcare marketing,
- describe the importance of flexibility in managing innovation,
- discuss organization structure and its impact on innovation, and
- explain the interorganization relationship and its implication on innovation.

## Introduction

Healthcare is one of the most rapidly changing industries. In order for contemporary healthcare organizations to continually survive and attain a competitive edge over others, they have to be able to innovate. Innovations play a key role in the development of healthcare delivery as it is a major driving force in the quest to balance healthcare cost and quality and enhance life expectancy, quality of life, and diagnostic and treatment options (Varkey, Horne & Bennet, 2008). Healthcare organizations' ability to innovate is often linked to the ideas of social networks within and between organizations. Innovation forms part of the system that produces it. A healthcare firm's ability to adopt an innovation is a prerequisite for the effective employment of new technologies and new inventions. On the other hand, healthcare organizations that adopt innovation are faced with difficulties and complicated opportunities, resulting in the need for new organizational procedures and the modification of managerial procedures. Technological and organizational innovations are intertwined. New markets, organizational modifications, novel procedures, and products are seen as elements of creative destructions (Schumpeter, 1950). Broadly, the adoption and manufacturing of a behavior or thought that is novel, as far as the healthcare organization is concerned, is referred to as organizational innovation (Damanpour, 1996).

## Uncertainty in Healthcare Institutions

Several changes are taking place in the healthcare delivery system. It is of utmost importance that healthcare firms that adopt innovation as a tool for continuous survival and growth try, as much as possible, to lessen uncertainties to the barest minimum, especially at those "critical" decision points. For example, it is very essential that in the effort to introduce a new product into the market, considerable uncertainty regarding consumers' reaction is reduced. However, it may be the case that some healthcare organizations may be faced with unfamiliar technological and marketing challenges and, therefore, assume an "entrepreneurial" stance with the supposition that some uncertainties may largely be uncontrollable.

An example of an initial interpretation of uncertainty is exemplified by Knight (1921) who differentiated between "risk," explained as an unfamiliar element to which chances can be apportioned, and "uncertainty," which are risks to which such chances cannot be apportioned. Nonetheless, even though the notion of uncertainty is prevalent in organizational studies, there is still no common conceptualization of the subject (Gales & Mansour-Cole, 1995). For instance, Galbraith (1977) has curiously posited that a great deal of uncertainty exists about the concept of uncertainty. Thus, uncertainty is interpreted with respect to information that necessitates action. From Galbraith's (1977) perspective, uncertainty implies the gap between the information needed to perform a task and information already possessed by the organization. Similarly, it has been claimed that uncertainty occurs when "details of situations are ambiguous and complex; when information is unavailable or inconsistent; and when people feel insecure about their own knowledge or the state of knowledge in general." Uncertainty can broadly be categorized into two, and these are discussed next:

## Technical Uncertainty

Generally, technical uncertainty is explained as the inability to foresee the nature of technical hitches which may occur in the course of development. Usually, these technical hitches require new technical solutions, which of course lead to the bloating of the initially projected cost.

## Market Uncertainty

Market uncertainty refers to the doubt regarding competing technologies, whether or not they impede the desire for innovation is being developed with feedback from consumers in mind as well as the likely market size for the product.

## Managing Uncertainty in Healthcare Institutions

There are several ways a healthcare institution can manage uncertainties in innovative business decision-making (Trott, 2008), and these are discussed next.

First, there should be employment of analytic tools that do not necessitate high precision since less sophisticated statistical tools are usually more reliable when it comes to managing complicated circumstances as compared to more sophisticated ones. The difficulty with more complicated tools is that they may fit previous data, but may be unable to envisage the future, whereas a simple tool may not fit previous data, but may possibly envisage the future.

Second, healthcare marketers should try to make several predictions instead of trying to make one accurate prediction, as this is how any true innovation functions. They should attach several small predictions to several possibilities.

Third, discover and depend on the foreseeable attributes of the circumstance.

Fourth, healthcare marketers should channel their energy towards the assessment of the creativity of innovation efforts and not just the outcome. Fifth, healthcare marketers need to be swift. They should make every effort to react fast. Nothing can replace the ability to spot events on time and stay attentive at all times. Healthcare organizations should lay emphasis on "sense and respond" and authorize their staff to react in a rapid and conclusive manner.

## Organizational Structure and Innovations

An organizational structure is a framework that traces how certain activities are guided to accomplish the objectives of a firm. These activities can incorporate guidelines, roles, and obligations. The organizational structure, likewise, decides how information streams from one level to another level within the organization. For instance, in a decision structure, choices spill out from the top–down, while in a decentralized structure, the choices are made at different levels/dimensions.

Organizational structure characterizes an explicit hierarchy within an organization. An effective organizational structure characterizes every representative's activity and how it fits within the general framework. This structuring gives an organization a visual portrayal of how it is formed and how it can best push ahead in accomplishing its objectives.

Organizations can be recognized by various qualities; for example, by the dissemination of power, by the multifaceted nature of the task structure and by motivating incentive frameworks. Wilson (1965), characterizes the structure as "the entirety of all rewards given to individuals," and makes what he calls *diversity* in an organization a key element and the likelihood of development action occurring at any of the phases of the inventive procedure. This element, diversity, is identifiable in the *task structure* and *incentive framework* in the organization. Wilson, at that point, hypothesizes three speculations: (a) "the greater the diversity of the organization the greater the likelihood that individuals will imagine significant advancements"; (b) "the more prominent the diversity of the organization, the greater the likelihood that real developments will be proposed"; and (c) "the more prominent the diversity of the organization, the smaller the extent of major imaginative recommendations that will be embraced."

The diversity qualities of associations as characterized by Wilson appear to correspond or be a close enough estimate to Weber's bureaucratic association framework, when diversity is low; and to a democratic or freestyle organization, when diversity is high. One may infer some valuable conclusions with respect to the structure of organizations and development. The freestyle organization where "everyone is required to work and co-work in a joint effort" is most appropriate for the commencement phase of advancement, while the bureaucratic organization appears to be indispensable in the adoption and usage stages.

Burns and Stalker (1961) were the first to demonstrate that different kinds of organizational structures may be viable in different circumstances. They recognize two extraordinary sorts of organizational structure: the mechanistic structure, which is found in organizations working under stable conditions and the natural structure, which is found, or rather is most appropriate, in associations working under/in insecure conditions. In clarifying why associations do not change their structure from mechanistic to natural when circumstances warrant it, Burns and Stalker underscore the role of resistance to change. They show that the political and status structures in the association may be compromised as the association changes and turns out to be progressively natural and amenable to manage developments. Changing from one type of association to the next tends to be seen from the attributes recognized, that everyone can turn into a potential source of contention. For instance, as the association turns out to be increasingly natural, there is more dispersion in decision-making. The general population that needs to give space for this to occur are probably going to set up resistance to safeguard their positions, subsequently making conflict.

Lawrence and Lorsch (1976) have shown that diverse parts of the association might be distinctive kinds of structures. Duncan (1973) goes above and beyond by demonstrating that the decision unit in the association may actualize distinctive types of organizational structures at various points in time. Duncan conceptualizes and measures structure regarding five measurements: hierarchy of power, level of unoriginality in decision-making, degree of participation in decision-making, level of explicit guidelines and systems, and level of division of work. Duncan, at that point, connects the summed-up idea of association to that of information and communication. He sees the association as a communication network held together by the stream of information. At the point when these measurements are very organized, channels of communication and measure of information accessibility are limited. By connecting the measure of information required at each point in time with the dimension of uncertainty in the environment, Duncan demonstrates that when information requests are low, a decision unit inside an association can react more rapidly to its environment by depending on preset guidelines and techniques, a very much determined division of work, amongst others. This may prevent the unit from looking for new sources of information, which may not have been predicted when the rules and procedures were originally established.

According to Kimberley and Evanisko (1981), environmental, individual, and organizational effects on innovation have been examined by several scholars. Notably, however, Robertson and Wind (1980) have posited that the choice of innovation by a firm is determined by certain organizational characteristics. Organizational innovativeness (Morrisson, 1996), firm size (Kennedy, 1983), and firm structure (Zaltman, Duncan & Holbek, 1973) have been recognized as the three kinds of characteristics that influence adoption at the organizational level. The inclination to adopt has been recurrently impacted by size. The adoption of innovation is often seen as having a positive relation to size. The reason mostly given is that, in order to enhance their performance, larger healthcare firms are inclined to adopt innovations. Interestingly, however, it can also be contended that smaller firms tend to be more innovative and adaptable because their smaller sizes make them more agile than larger firms. We argue that for healthcare institutions, the degree to which an organization is receptive to new products or ideas will influence its propensity to adopt new products. Therefore, firms will probably channel their efforts towards innovation if they put in place strategies that are innovation inclined and competitive.

## Flexibility

When Duncan (1976) spoke of the ambidextrous model, he implied flexibility. Thereafter, the word *ambidextrous* was employed in illustrating firms that were able to initiate complete and gradual modifications grounded on the congruency amid individuals, culture, and structure (Tushman & O'Really, 1996). For instance, healthcare firms that are capable of introducing new products, by adopting flexible structures, will arguably be ahead of their competition (Miles & Snow 1986). A more specific formulation of the relationship between flexibility and innovation is made by Sanchez and McKinley (1998), and this refers to both structural flexibility and the production process. The former is measured in terms of the "youthfulness" of the organization, considering that more elderly organizations may possess strong structural inertia which will have a negative influence upon flexibility. The latter is measured in terms of *customization* or *product flexibility* (Vickery, Calantone, & Droge, 1999), because when a company reaches an agreement with the specifications of a client, it becomes necessary to make investments which will facilitate the necessary modifications to the production processes. This attribute will have to be based upon a redefining of the roles and responsibilities, which must be widely adopted and which are considered to be one of the principles of the design of innovative healthcare organizations (Dougherty 1992). This creates the context makes the generation and exploitation of knowledge possible.

## Communication

One other remarkable attribute of healthcare firms that is innovative is their systems of communications. Fundamentally, the notion is that when procedures are made too formal, it may impede the development of innovative solutions within the healthcare organization (Von Hippel, 1998). Innovative healthcare organizations must, therefore, have routines at their disposal that can cut across any limits established by the organizational structure (Pitt & Clark, 1999). This implies significant adaptations of the classical use of data as an origin of controlled, inadequate authority and can be translated into a tool that improves upon efficacy and is broadcasted all throughout the healthcare firm and made electronically accessible (Daft & Lewin, 1993). New technologies have effectively changed the way communication is done and have, in some cases, led to the development of "virtual work teams," where a number of persons positioned at different locations can communicate effectively through video conferencing, the internet, or intranet (Hitt, Keats, & De Marie, 1998) to solve critical health issues.

## Interorganizational Relationships

Not only is communication broadening, but it is also becoming uninterrupted within the boundaries of healthcare organizations. One of the aspects related to organizational design, which has taken on greater significance in the recent past, is associated with the increased blurring of organizational networks through strategic alliances. The flow of information is, therefore, not limited to functions within an organization, but also between customers, suppliers, designers, and other firms as well. This is of great significance as far as innovation is concerned because, it facilitates concurrent experimentation of new initiatives, thereby, leading to a rapid learning process. Interorganizational information flow is also a characteristic of these interorganizational relationships.

Innovation is essential for the long-term prosperity and growth of the healthcare organization, especially in dynamic markets. It can be argued that the imaginative capability of a healthcare institution resides in the knowledge, aptitudes, and capacities of its employees. Healthcare institutions need to develop mechanisms to distinguish the attributes and practices of innovative individuals and advance and energize such individuals within the healthcare institutional organization.

## Conclusion

The uncertainty in healthcare institutions was presented, suggesting the need for a healthcare provider to be more innovative and to meet the ever-changing needs of their customers and the industry. For contemporary healthcare organizations to continually survive and attain a competitive edge over others, they must be able to innovate. Healthcare organizations' ability to innovate is often linked to the ideas of social networks within and between organizations. Innovation forms part of the system that produces it.

Innovations should be flexible and adaptable. It may warrant the need to redefine roles and responsibilities within the organization, this, however, must be effectively communicated. The organization must ensure that stakeholders are motivated to engage with the innovation. Stakeholders, including staff, should be aware of the whole process, aware of expectations, and be supported through the process. If need be, there should be training and public awareness to develop the interorganization relationship and make everyone conversant with the changes and capable of adapting to them.

The flow of information is, therefore, not limited to functions within an organization, but also between customers, suppliers, designers, and other firms as well. This is of great significance as far as innovation is concerned, because it facilitates concurrent experimentation of new initiatives, thereby, leading to a rapid learning process. Interorganizational information flow is also a characteristic of these interorganizational relationships.

## Review Questions

1. Explain how innovations can be communicated in the context of healthcare marketing.
2. Describe the importance of flexibility in managing innovation.
3. Discuss organizational structure and its impact on innovation.

### MINI CASE STUDY: INNOVATION—WELLNESS APP

The 15-year-old Anastasia Health System (AHS) has a clientele base of 750 hospitals and over 100 health centers. Its staff strength is over 10,000, with more than 1,000 affiliated medical doctors. Their primary goal is to deliver healthcare services to meet the health needs of their target market, including distribution of medical equipment, products, and prescriptions.

To diversify its services, AHS recently developed the I-Relax app designed to help health-conscious people do three things:

1. track diet and exercise;
2. monitor blood sugar levels and blood pressure; and
3. find doctors, read real reviews, and book appointments instantly.

Using I-Relax, patients are now able to monitor their health status on the go. Data trends from patients' continuous usage facilitate a follow-up response from a pharmacist, a doctor, or even a health coach. The success of the I-Relax app has led to the introduction of several other technology-driven platforms targeted at specific health issues. These new programs seem to be working well, and users are happy.

The management of AHS was concerned that their novel health-tracking app, I-Relax, had not generated quick returns on investment and were reluctant to continue to fund such technology. However, being innovative is part of their brand proposition, and the company was gradually being known as a leader in healthcare and technology.

### Discussion Questions

1. Should AHS continue with the app at a loss, or develop other programs that may be financially sustainable? Is launching a

marketing campaign for I-Relax going to attract users, or should AHS limit its distribution to specific clientele just as they would do with other medical products or prescriptions?

2. For the product to be profitable, AHS must expand its market share. What marketing strategies can be put in place to increase visibility, improve market share, and ensure the profitability of an innovative product?

## References

Burns, T., & Stalker, G. M. (1961). *The management of innovation.* London, England: Tavistock.

Daft, R. L., & Lewin, A. Y. (1993). Where are the theories for the" new" organizational forms? An editorial essay. *Organization Science,* i–vi.

Damanpour, F. (1996). Organizational complexity and innovation: Developing and testing multiple contingency models. *Management Science, 42*(5), 693–716.

Dougherty, D. (1992). Interpretive barriers to successful product innovation in large firms. *Organization Science, 3*(2), 179–202.

Duncan, R. B. (1976). The ambidextrous organization: Designing dual structures for innovation. *The Management of Organization: Strategy and Implementation, 1,* 167–188.

Duncan, Z. H. (1973). *Innovations and organizations.* Hoboken, NJ: Wiley.

Galbraith, J. R. (1977). *Organization design.* New York, NY: Addison Wesley.

Gales, L., & Mansour-Cole, D. (1995). User involvement in innovation projects: Toward an information processing model. *Journal of Engineering and Technology Management, 12*(1–2), 77–109.

Hitt, M. A., Keats, B. W., & DeMarie, S. M. (1998). Navigating in the new competitive landscape: Building strategic flexibility and competitive advantage in the 21st century. *Academy of Management Perspectives, 12*(4), 22–42.

Kennedy, A. M. (1983). The adoption and diffusion of new industrial products: A literature review. *European Journal of Marketing, 17*(3), 31–88.

Kimberly, J. R., & Evanisko, M. J. (1981). Organizational innovation: The influence of individual, organizational, and contextual factors on hospital adoption of technological and administrative innovations. *Academy of Management Journal, 24*(4), 689–713.

Knight, F. H. (1921). Cost of production and price over long and short periods. *Journal of Political Economy, 29*(4), 304–335.

Lawrence, P. R., & Lorsch, J. W. (1976). *Organization and environment.* Cambridge, MA: Mass. Management of Innovation.

Miles, R. E., & Snow, C. C. (1986). Organizations: New concepts for new forms. *California Management Review, 28*(3), 62–73.

Morrisson, P. (1996). *Testing a framework for the adoption of technological innovations by organizations and the role of leading edge users.* University Park, PA: Institute for the Study of Business Markets Report.

Pitt, M., & Clarke, K. (1999). Competing on competence: A knowledge perspective on the management of strategic innovation. *Technology Analysis & Strategic Management, 11*(3), 301–316.

Robertson, T. S., & Wind, Y. (1980). Organizational psychographics and innovativeness. *Journal of Consumer Research, 7*(1), 24–31.

Sanchez, C. M., & McKinley, W. (1998). Environmental regulatory influence and product innovation: The contingency effects of organizational characteristics. *Journal of Engineering and Technology Management, 15*(4), 257–278.

Schumpeter, J. A. (1950). *Capitalism, socialism, and democracy* (3rd ed.). New York, NY: Harper & Row.

Trott, P. (2008). *Innovation management and new product development.* London, England: Pearson Education.

Tushman, M. L., & O'Really, C. H. (1996). Ambidextros organizations: Managing evolutionary and revolutionary change. *California Management Review, 38*(4), 8–30.

Varkey, P., Horne, A., & Bennet, K. E. (2008). Innovation in health care: A primer. *American Journal of Medical Quality, 23*(5), 382–388.

Vickery, S. N., Calantone, R., & Droge, C. (1999). Supply chain flexibility: An empirical study. *Journal of supply chain management, 35*(2), 16–24.

Von Hippel, E. (1998). Economics of product development by users: The impact of "sticky" local information. *Management Science, 44*(5), 629–644.

Wilson, J. Q. (1965). *Innovation in organization: Notes toward a theory.* New York, NY: Center for the Advanced Study of Educational Administration.

Zaltman, G., Duncan, R., & Holbek, J. (1973). *Innovations and organizations.* New York, NY: Wiley.

# 7

## *Healthcare Stakeholders*

### Chapter Outline

- Introduction
- Who is a Stakeholder?
- Stakeholders in Healthcare Sector
- Stakeholder Theory
- Stakeholder Value
- Difference Between a Stakeholder and a Shareholder
- Stakeholder Identification
- Generic Stakeholder Identification
- Engagement Guidelines
- Snowballing
- Mapping
- Identifying Stakeholders' Needs
- Managing Value Through Stakeholder Management
- Sustaining Stakeholder Value
- Managing Sustainable Stakeholder Value
- Conclusion
- Review Questions
- Mini Case Study With Discussion Questions
- References

*Marketing in Healthcare-Related Industries*, pages 145–171
Copyright © 2020 by Information Age Publishing
**145**

## Chapter Outcome

By the end of this chapter, the reader will be able to

- explain who stakeholders are,
- explain the stakeholder value approach,
- understand how health sector stakeholders can be identified, and
- understand how value is created for stakeholders in the health sector.

## Introduction

In this chapter, the book treats one of the key concepts of relevance to healthcare marketing: stakeholders management, particularly in a competitive and dynamic environment. In contemporary times, the healthcare environment has become progressively competitive. The small hospital or health facility needs to market itself just as the larger and well-known ones. However, the approach to marketing by these differing entities may vary greatly. In modern times, even monopolistic public sector organizations realize that they have to stay relevant and maintain customer satisfaction and ensure high morale among their employees. The stakeholders of a specialist fertility clinic may be markedly different from a teaching hospital. An academic medical center can emphasize education, research, or community service and have patient care as a secondary function (Thomas, 2008). Different healthcare institutions carry different stakeholder constituencies, and thus, for marketing to be successfully carried out, there is the need to delve into stakeholder needs and how to deliver value to stakeholders.

Stakeholders throughout the healthcare marketing process are crucial because success and the continual existence of public health institutions, for example, hinge on meeting key stakeholder demands according to how they interpret value (Bryson, 2004; Moore, 1995). Most healthcare organizations are chartered as not-for-profit organizations. This not-for-profit orientation has differentiated the healthcare sector from other industries. As a result, marketers who have operated mainly in other sectors rather than in healthcare may marvel at how healthcare institutions usually enthusiastically engage in services that may not lead to making a profit. Another reason for the dynamism of the healthcare sector is the government support operators receive in the sector. As contended by Rainey (1999), public agencies (like public not-for-profit hospitals) survive by ensuring that their activities satisfy stakeholders and lead to the sustenance of the agencies' political legitimacy and the resources attached. So, for example, if the main stakeholders are unsatisfied, at least insignificantly, with respect to their standards for satisfaction, usually, the belief is that there should be some adaptations. When stakeholders are satisfied, they reward organizations with resources and withdraw resources when they are unsatisfied.

## Who Is a Stakeholder?

The initial interpretation of a stakeholder by Freeman (1984) is usually attributed to an internal report from the Stanford Research Institute (SRI) in 1963. Stakeholders were elucidated as "those groups without whose support the healthcare organization would cease to exist" (Fontaine, Haarman, & Schmid, 2006). This interpretation was adapted by Freeman (2004) as "those groups who are vital to the survival and success of the organization." Freeman's organizationally inclined interpretation where the author defines stakeholders as "any group or individual who can affect or is affected by the achievement of the healthcare organization objectives," is preferred by scholars and is regularly used. Most of the definitions are in line with this interpretation. According to Friedman and Miles (2006), this definition is more composed and far-reaching as compared to the interpretation given by SRI. The phrase "can affect or is affected by" appears to embrace entities outside the firm and groups. A common way of distinguishing amongst several kinds of stakeholders is to examine classes of individuals who have relationships (with organizations) that are capable of being grouped. Friedman and Miles (2006) implies that there is a distinct connection within interpretations of "What are stakeholders?" and identification of "Who are the stakeholders?"

## Stakeholders in Healthcare Sector

The key stakeholders in the healthcare system include patients, providers, payers, and policymakers. There are many other individuals and groups, including government, employers, and pharmaceutical companies involved in the healthcare system who have their own economic interests to protect. These stakeholders could have a positive or negative influence on the marketing efforts of healthcare institutions if they are not managed properly.

### *Consumers/Patients*

These refer to those individuals with the potential to consume healthcare service. Evidently, at some point in life, everyone will most likely utilize healthcare services. Increasingly, patients are becoming involved in making healthcare choices as their burden of healthcare costs continues to grow (Corbin, Kelley, & Schwartz, 2001). They are becoming more informed consumers, and their expectations of healthcare services continue to rise as a result. For the demand for state-of-the-art technological services, new prescription drugs, and expensive treatments will continue to escalate. The old healthcare model is primarily driven by the medical model, which focuses on illness rather than wellness, but the current healthcare model increasingly emphasizes disease prevention, wellness promotion, early intervention, and illness management. In several developing countries, the most common healthcare services that individuals receive is from pharmaceutical firms through purchases of over-the-counter drugs. Others also purchase items such as self-help books, fitness equipment, and health food, among others. This causes the healthcare sector to have varied consumers.

### Family and Relatives

Family members often play important roles in managing chronic illnesses, choosing healthcare providers, and treatment of patients. While some customers may be able to voice their concerns, parents and relatives of customers are also considered stakeholders. This is particularly as relates to the vulnerable adults and children, parents and relatives are involved in their care and can, therefore, act in the best interest of their family member. They want to make sure quality healthcare is being provided; they can decide to transfer their family member to another hospital if they believe adequate care is not being offered.

### Clinical Personnel

These are usually physicians and other clinicians as well. They are medically trained to provide healthcare. These are doctors, dentists, nurses, and other clinical professionals. Physicians play a key role in the healthcare system, as they constitute a significant share of demand for health services and are directly or indirectly responsible for most healthcare expenditures (Thomas, 2004). Primary care physicians serve as gatekeepers who diagnose and treat illnesses and injuries and refer patients to medical specialists if this is determined to be appropriate. Their training and the quality of the care they provide have a visible effect on the patients, as well as on the hospital where the diagnosis or treatment takes place. Physicians and dentists also deal with any applicable insurance companies and government programs, as well as with the vendors and suppliers who deal with their clinic or private practice. Although most of the day-by-day care of patients in hospitals is provided by nurses, they usually are only allowed to provide the treatment that is decided upon by the physician. However, in the setting of a healthcare organization, the goals and objectives of these clinical professionals may vary from that of the administrators of the organization. The operations of these health professionals are guided by medical ethics, which has no bearing on the operation of the organization as a system. Therefore, health professionals may make medical decisions that are in the best interest of the patient, but may not bring in profits to the health organization.

## Nonclinical Personnel

It is essential to also recognize the role of nonclinical personnel within the stakeholder structure of healthcare provision. They are often described as support staff, and they include the employees of the IT department, accounts, and the procurement and marketing team. They are different from contractors as they are employed by the organization, often in a full-time position. They are not responsible for the hands-on healthcare provision because they have not been medically trained, but they provide the background work end support. Porters, cleaners, drivers, and healthcare assistants also fall in this category. They can also be members of trade unions or trade associations.

## Health Insurance Companies

Insurance companies are major players in the healthcare system. They function as intermediaries between patients and providers. Insurance agencies/managed care organizations (MCOs) and government programs employ various mechanisms for insuring against risk. They market a wide variety of healthcare insurance plans directly to patients or indirectly through employers or governmental intermediaries. Health insurance premiums (the amount charged by the insurer to insure against risk) vary by numerous factors, including types of plan, age of insured, as well as geographical location. Access to healthcare services may be selectively based on insurance coverage. Insurance companies are criticized for raising premiums and refusing medical coverage for certain conditions.

## Administrators

Although managers/administrators hold a great stake in healthcare organizations, many scholars have differing opinions about whether they should be classified as stakeholders. While some see them as stakeholders, others see them as symbols of the organization's responsibilities and actions.

Notably, Aoki (1984) conceptualizes managers as mediators between employees and financiers who may regard themselves as stakeholders of an organization without the firm seeing them as such. The administrators are responsible for the strategic direction of the organization. They liaise with the stakeholders, shareholders, and regulators. They oversee the day-to-day administrative operations including planning, coordination, and supervision of facilities and human resources. They may have started their career as clinical or nonclinical personnel, as they understand the sector and can, therefore, provide strategic leadership. They make decisions and are responsible for the outcomes. If things go wrong strategically, for example, if the financial targets are not being met, they are more likely to be sacked than other personnel. Since the healthcare industry is undergoing a variety of changes, healthcare administrators face unique challenges.

### Contractors

These stakeholders are not necessarily employed by the organization, but they provide services to ensure the smooth running of the organization and this also ensures a quality service. They include the suppliers of clinical goods who expects to be paid in time for their deliveries, waste disposal agents for companies that are responsible for clinical waste, power and water suppliers to make sure the organization has the basic utilities to operate. If these contractors are not well catered for, they can disrupt the smooth running of the organization.

### Allied Service Providers

These are stakeholders that provide services that are needed to complete the healthcare provision. They are not specifically owned or contracted by the health organizations as they also have their own vested interest. These include the health insurance companies who may want their clients to use a hospital because they can arrange a better deal. There are those who organize health tourism and visit overseas countries for those who may not be able to get the needed treatment in their own country. These also include media, advertising, and public relation agencies that focus on the health sector, creating contents for the health sector to engage with the customers.

### Financiers

These are those with vested financial interest in the organization. The success of the organization guarantees a high yield for their investments.

They are shareholders who have invested in the organization and they want the organization to do well. This is quite common in the private healthcare sectors where investment has been made in facilities and staffs to attract customers who can pay for premium care. Other financiers, other than stakeholders, include debt holders, bondholders, and creditors.

## Community

Unlike the private health sector where there are financiers who have invested in the organization, the public sector has its community as a stakeholder. Members of a local society will always want a healthcare center within their community. They want access to healthcare, and they have vested interest in the running of the organization, making sure it is well run and managed. They are more likely to be the main target audience for marketing activities and patronage for the organization.

## Government Agencies and Regulators

Government plays an important role in healthcare as it is the single largest payer of healthcare expenditure in many countries. In a country that has a publicly funded national healthcare system, the government even manages the infrastructure for the delivery of medical care. Healthcare is regulated, and it is not surprising that organizations are expected to be operated based on laid down ethical guidelines and regulations. Government agencies like the Ministry of Health are key stakeholders in healthcare policy and provision, especially in liberal democratic nations. They can enforce laws and government rulings; they make sure the organization is run by competent and qualified individuals. If this is not adhered to, it can affect the reputation of the organization, and the organization might even be shut down. Other agencies such as advertising regulators might also be involved to ensure that advertisements are not making misleading medical claims. Health insurance regulators are also interested in managing customers, using their insurance in the organization, to make sure they are receiving the treatment they deserve. In the United States, the Federal Trade Commission (FTC) is responsible for overseeing and regulating advertising and other marketing-related communications. Pharmaceutical marketing and its ethical aspects have long been a subject of debate with regard to traditional media, and promotion of prescription drugs through electronic media, which poses even greater ethical challenges (Huhmann & Limbu, 2016). Thus, the Office of Prescription Drug Promotion (OPDP), a division of the FDA, issues guidelines and oversees the advertising of prescription drug products in the United States.

The FDA issues warnings and untitled letters to pharmaceutical marketers for violations of regulations that have mostly resulted from the omission or lack of risk information, misleading/false claims, omission of material facts, and labeling issues (Limbu, McKinley, & Temperini, 2019).

---

### *Pharmaceutical Companies*

Pharmaceutical companies play an important role in the healthcare system because they sell their products to patients. The pharmaceutical market is bound to play a crucial role in the future of healthcare, both in terms of quality of life and cost. Spending on prescription drugs has been cited as a leading contributor to the increase in overall health spending. The prices for drugs are rising globally; drugs makers have faced intense pressure to lower prices. An increasingly large percentage of prescriptions are written for branded drugs. Many physicians' prescribing behaviors are influenced by their meetings with pharmaceutical sales representatives.

## Stakeholder Theory

The stakeholder theory is grounded in the belief that "the firm takes into account all of those groups and individuals that can affect, or are affected by, the accomplishment of organizational purpose" (Freeman, 1984). Managers can no longer be responsible only for activities that will ensure a profit for the healthcare organization, but must participate in activities that will render the organization socially responsible and, thus, seek ways to satisfy their key stakeholders (Savage, Nix, Whitehead, & Blair, 1991). Mitchell, Agle, and Wood (1997) posit that the salience of stakeholders should be identified by managers based on the degree to which they give priority to stakeholder claims and argue that managers must attend to power and urgency, as some stakeholders exhibit certain attributes in order to serve the legal and moral interests of legitimate stakeholders.

The stakeholder theory, when applied to healthcare marketing activity, would normally task marketing managers to ask themselves the following questions: Are any stakeholders being unfairly or unjustly affected by marketing activities? Are their ethical and legal claims being recognized, discussed, and addressed by the healthcare marketing organization? For healthcare marketing managers who profess that ethical concerns are central to the building of trust among stakeholders, it is these questions that require greater reflection and ultimately shape how microlevel transactions in particular market segments should be assessed from a macro or public policy standpoint.

The premise of an individual or group having a "stake" in a healthcare organization can be broadly defined. On the one hand, a stakeholder might have a legal claim on the organization, for example, owners who expect a certain level of financial performance. In another case, a stakeholder, such as the general public, may just be concerned with how the healthcare organization influences the country's economic growth. As can be seen from the examples, stakeholder prominence can differ, just as the precise organizational issues they are concerned with can differ. Hence, employing the stakeholder theory to the development of marketing objectives is an exceptionally multifaceted procedure.

A hard-form stakeholder theory advocates that the purpose of the healthcare organization is much broader than merely achieving customer satisfaction at the firm level or wealth maximization for the company's shareholders. Understandably, both these elements are (and should be) part of the guiding doctrine of almost all healthcare marketing firms. However, the purpose of health businesses (writ large), from the standpoint of stakeholder theory, goes beyond the micro-firm level, and the aim is to help promote the greater common good of the stakeholder network, collectively. The hard-form stakeholder theory posits that the creation of "value" by the firm is to be understood broadly and socially, not merely from the customer's and shareholder's perspectives (Freeman, Wicks, & Parmar, 2004).

## Stakeholder Value

Stakeholder valuing, as a real-world implementation of stakeholder theory, starts with the construction of identity and then moves to outlining and assessing the value of individual stakeholders (groups). A firm starts the process of valuing its stakeholders by following Brickson's recommendation (2005) and first tries to ask the question: What is our relationship with the stakeholder and what is the stakeholder's relationship with us? Brickson (2005) proposes that the response to this question may be classified under three broad categories: independent, dyadically independent, or derived from group membership. Healthcare organizations that have independent relationships have individualistic inclinations and, hence, do not generally attach more value to stakeholders. Healthcare organizations that are dyadically independent or have relational orientations tend to place a higher value on some stakeholder groups than others. Healthcare organizations that have collectivist inclinations/orientations form their identities from group members, as they see all groups as valuable. This is imperative in valuing stakeholders since the identities motivate the firm's driving factors.

Brickson (2005) recommends that the main inspiring element for independent firms is utilitarian, that is, the organization is mostly interested in its well-being. Their (independent firms') main aim is profit, even though the motives for the goal may differ. Dyadically independent firms are basically utilitarian in nature but acknowledge that their victory hinges heavily on relationships with a number of important stakeholders, specifically on the customers. Brickson (2005) submits that several service organizations are seen as dyadically independent organizations as their success relies heavily on their clients, and as such, some of their identity is formed by those clients. This means that the reputation or image of a professional service firm could be enhanced by having some kind of businesses as clients. Since the identities differ, the entries on the balance sheet will also differ, sometimes noticeably, from organization to organization, considering the value attached to various stakeholders by the firm and how this value is communicated to shareholders as well as other stakeholders.

Academics who accentuate the theory of identity creation (Brickson, 2005, 2007; Bundi, Shropsphire, Buchholt, 2013) contend that an organization's identity and stakeholder valuing are indivisibly connected. An organization's identity is a social construction emanating from relations within the organization, as symbolized by its managers, and its several stakeholder groups (Scott & Lane, 2000). In support of this, Brickson (2005) constructs identity creation on what the author terms the *descriptive branch* of the stakeholder theory, proposing that it is through this standpoint that the stakeholder theory can "help reinstate a balanced perspective of the firm" by advancing both the contributory and normative consequences of the diverse methods to the stakeholder theory. A principal benefit of this viewpoint is that it "moves us away from a discussion about whether organizations should engage with stakeholders to a view in which all organizations do actively engage with stakeholders, but in very different ways, each with potential to create distinct forms of social value" (Brickson, 2007, p. 866). With regards to individuals, an organization's identity can be widely classified as individualistic, relational, or collectivist. Individualistic identity inclinations are characteristically interpretations of independence—how the organization is distinct from other organizations with their own well-being as the main driving force in decision-making. Relational orientations are opinions of interdependence within the setting of linking with specific others, assuring that their well-being is the main instigator. A collectivist orientation is a "greater good" standpoint with an emphasis on the welfare of the group as a whole.

However, these classifications are not mutually exclusive. Instead, Brickson (2007) suggests that a firm's identity consists of a combination of traits from each of the three categories. Brickson (2005) declares that organizations can have diverse types of interactions with diverse stakeholders and that firm-level variables are the interpreters of those associations. These variables include the firm's industry, the type of customer/client that the firm serves, the firm's size, and the age of the firm (Brickson, 2007).

## Difference Between a Stakeholder and a Shareholder

It is important to note that in the public sector, more of the dealings are with stakeholders. The public sector mostly comprises of state corporations which do not primarily have shareholders. However, it is still important to know the differences between stakeholders and shareholders, who give money to a company to be a part owner of the company by buying stocks or a portion of the company. This is of great importance to the company as it helps to raise a reasonable amount of capital for the company. At the other end, shareholders get their own share of benefits from the company's profit, depending on how much the company earns. However, because of their part ownership of the company through shares, shareholders are considered the most important stakeholders of the company. This is because the dealings, fortunes, and misfortunes of the company will have a direct impact on them. For instance, shareholders will share in the profits made by the company through dividends. Should the company make losses, then the shareholders will bear the consequences of such.

The other stakeholders of the company may have a direct or indirect interest in the company. Stakeholders are people that are affected by the positive or negative happenings of a company. Examples of stakeholders include customers, suppliers, employees and their families, among others. Shareholders are also examples of stakeholders. This is because of the direct impact the firm's successes, and failures have on them. Some organizations can only have stakeholders and no shareholders. An example of this is a typical public university. Public universities do not float shares as they are mainly owned by the government. Therefore, they have no shareholders. However, these public universities have several stakeholders. The stakeholders of public universities include teachers, students, administrators, janitors, and suppliers of stationery.

## Stakeholder Identification

According to Freeman (2010), examining stakeholders helps institutions to identify and classify their stakeholders. Despite the fact that not all stakeholders have a key stake in decisions or policy-making, there may be the need to identify all stakeholders (Donaldson & Preston, 1995), and it is noteworthy to identify stakeholders before they are ranked (Rawlins, 2006) since their stakes, impacts, and power may change over time (Achterkamp & Vos, 2007). Stakeholders may also have numerous roles, and a number of stakeholders may play the same role (Ballejos & Montagna, 2008). Appropriate identification of stakeholders is important for a firm's success (Achterkamp & Vos, 2008).

Scholars have come out with four distinct key methods for identifying stakeholders. These are the use of a generic list, asking a set of questions, using the snowballing technique, and stakeholder mapping (Mathur, Price, Austin, & Moobela, 2007). The first three methods are techniques in identifying stakeholders, while stakeholder mapping serves as a strategic approach in connection to the planning and designing of the successive engagement approach. Otherwise stated, mapping stakeholders can commence during the initial stages through to the last stages of the stakeholder identification process where appropriate techniques are selected and utilized.

## Generic Stakeholder Identification

It is helpful to initiate the stakeholder identification process by first considering identifying the conventional stakeholder groups and types in a specific setting. Table 7.1 summarizes the broad stakeholder types as indicated by the three primary categories of stakeholders: those who affect the project, those who are affected by the project, and others who may be interested. It ought to be noted that some stakeholders may belong to more than one category; they may influence the project and be influenced by it as well. The following grouping is beneficial in the beginning, to list the names of organizations or identify the individuals who should be considered for engagement.

## Engagement Guidelines

Mostly, engagement guidelines propose the use of a list of questions to ensure that every stakeholder is considered (English Nature, 2002; Mathur et al., 2007). Those involved in the delivery of a project must start by asking questions in order to identify the stakeholders. Some of these questions include the following:

- ▪ Who is accountable for the project?
- ▪ Who is accountable for statutory duties?
- ▪ Who benefits from the project?

| TABLE 7.1 | The Generic Stakeholder Categories and Types | |
|---|---|---|
| **Broad Category** | **Sub-Category** | **Types of Individuals/Groups** |
| Those who affect the project | Those involved in the delivery of the project | Developer |
| | | Client |
| | | Owner |
| | | Investor |
| | | Designer |
| | | Banks insurance |
| | | Professional consultants such as architectural, financial, structural, etc. |
| | Those who determine the context | Local authority-planning departments, etc. |
| | | Regional government departments |
| | | Central government departments |
| | | Non-departmental public bodies such as Environmental Agency, Housing Corporation, etc. |
| Those who are affected by the project | Directly affected | Users of the buildings, spaces, facilities, etc. |
| | May be directly or indirectly affected depending on the context | Local/surrounding community members |
| | | General public |
| | | Local community groups such as resident associations, or other community-based groups |
| | | Specific demographic groups such as those based on race, ethnicity, gender, age |
| Others who may be interested | | Environmental/social campaigning organizations |
| | | Research/academics |
| | | Media |
| | | Potential users/clients for future projects |

*Source:* Marthur, Price, Austin, & Moobela, 2007.

- Who are those affected by the business, but yet, voiceless?
- Who is likely to oppose the project and cause negative results?
- Who runs the organization with an intended positive mindset?
- Who can stand for the interest of those who cannot participate?
- Who is mandated to make decisions on behalf of those they represent?
- Who has unusually great ideas related to the project?
- Who has cultural or historical connections, related to the area or to any issues that the project raises?
- Who depends on the resources (natural or otherwise) which may be affected by the project? (Mathur et al., 2007)

Jennings and Lockie (2002) have underlined that there is a need to ensure that the belief of all the varied interests within the community is characterized by democratically elected politicians. This does not, however, prevent direct forms of involvement. By considering such questions, the team can help in ensuring that no stakeholder is neglected, and the list composed is adequately comprehensive.

## Snowballing

The moment these stakeholders have been recognized, they need to be called together for their views on who should be considered as important stakeholders. In other words, healthcare firms should adopt the snowballing technique to help them to identify these stakeholders and other members (Ananda & Herath, 2003; Hair, Bush, & Ortinau, 2000). Stakeholders' opinions in respect of whom they perceive as being stakeholders in the project may be obtained through focus group discussions, interviews, and questionnaires (Araujo & Bramwell, 1999). It has been adduced to be a relatively inexpensive and effective way of identifying the stakeholders (Ananda & Herath, 2003).

According to Hair et al. (2000), the snowballing technique may result in prejudices if there are substantial differences amid those groups who are recognized within established social circles and those who are not. It is likely that those potential stakeholders who are less distinctly visible may not be recognized, but that weakness can be overcome. It is suggested that there should be a mapping of the stakeholders identified through the snowballing method in order to begin designing the engagement, by recognizing the connection between them, resulting in the identification of stakeholders.

It has been emphasized that, while recognizing stakeholders, the concerns of any legitimate stakeholder should not be overlooked merely because they are not easy to identify in the planning of the project (Department for International Development, UK, 2002). This highlights the need for making sure that the stakeholders recognized can constitute the array of interests as well as interests of those who cannot be involved directly, particularly in terms of the key sustainability matters like intergenerational equity and global climate change.

## Mapping

Numerous stakeholders may have interests that are hidden, or others may have uncertain interests. Some interests of diverse stakeholders may also be in conflict with those of other people. It is imperative to find these interests at this phase so as to circumvent any real conflicts from developing in the evaluation process, which may be attained, for example, by involving certain stakeholders separately and in a distinct way instead of altogether in the same forum, if needed. Figure 7.1 shows the mapping of stakeholders based on their power or interest.

It is critical to comprehend the power that every stakeholder possesses, because it brings the emphasis on controlling or empowering the influence of the different stakeholders during the engagement. The diverse groups of stakeholders are viewed differently by scholars. For instance, stakeholders can be internal employees, managers, trade union members, departments, or they can be external customers, suppliers, or pressure group. Some scholars view stakeholders in terms of primary and secondary stakeholders. The primary stakeholders are stakeholders who define the business and are very important to the existence of an organization. Examples of primary stakeholders include suppliers, customers, investors in the community, and employee stakeholders. Again, secondary stakeholders are those stakeholders whose activities may have an effect on the activities of the primary stakeholders. For instance, pressure from the environment may have an influence on customers if there are allusions that products fail to meet the ecological standards. Aside from that, stakeholders also include consumer groups, inspectors, business partners, competitors, and regulators. A public sector contractor, for example, might list central or local government as a primary, rather than a secondary stakeholder. Another instance is that a train company or media company may list its industry regulator as a primary stakeholder. Now, being able to identify the various stakeholders, there is the basis to know their needs. Hence, the next section discusses the needs of stakeholders.

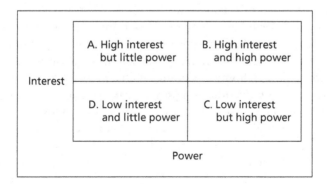

**Figure 7.1** Mapping stakeholders on a power/interest grid. *Source:* Derived from DFID, 2002.

## Identifying Stakeholders' Needs

Stakeholder needs can differ based on their relationship to the organization, that is, internal or external stakeholders. Thus this section discusses the various needs of categories of stakeholders.

### Internal Stakeholders' Needs Satisfaction

Internal stakeholders are those who work in an organization. This implies that internal stakeholders cannot be restricted to any one specific individual. As such, anybody within the firm from any of the departments can be an internal stakeholder. For example, internal stakeholders are made up of employees from functional units within the healthcare organization; it includes the manufacturing, marketing, and the research units of an organization. Employees knowing the principal requirements of their job within the organization find their work meaningful and to their satisfaction. This is followed by remuneration and acknowledgement of their efforts in the work they do. The reward (or pay) for work is fulfilling to employees when they judge it to be reasonable remuneration for their work. In such instances, reasonableness is a component of the individual's skills, efforts, quality, convictions, philosophy, and standards. Most workers make this judgment dependent on examinations with other individuals, both inside and outside their organization. It is a typical practice for business organizations to quantify the compensation rates of different organizations.

Several employees consider acknowledgment for work done to be as noteworthy as remuneration, that is, as long as their remuneration meets their needs. When employees perceive their remuneration to be inadequate, recognition may become important. There is nothing more fulfilling to an individual or a team than for an admired leader to appreciate good work done. However, even more important to employees is meaningful, challenging work. In conventional organizations, a typical misconception amongst managers and leaders is that some people just want to do the work, get paid, and go home. A significant challenge for leaders is to satisfy the hidden needs of individual employees. Meaningful work, regardless of whether recognized or not, is work that challenges employees' to be mentally, emotionally, and socially assertive. People want to engage in work that necessitates them to expend energy. There is nothing more destructive to the human condition than uninteresting, monotonous work. The best work performance systems are able to challenge workers to develop innovative competencies to help the organization achieve its strategic objectives. They additionally define objectives for workers that are measured in value-added terms: value-added for customers and society. This incorporates productivity measures, such as improvement of service delivery-time for customers; quality measures, such as the number of services offered within customers' specifications; and service measures, such as decrement in emissions and waste materials released into the environment.

### External Stakeholders' Needs Satisfaction

Several establishments regrettably make little effort to identify the needs and opinions of external stakeholders past the bare minimum. Thus, they only communicate with customers when required and do not go beyond to bond with their customers. Several establishments habitually disregard societal stakeholders, which include the communities around their facilities, plants, and offices. A few organizations are oblivious of the desires of their external stakeholders past the prerequisites of fulfilling either clients or the ego needs of the firm. Also, there are people beyond the customers and employees, namely the communities affected by these businesses. It must be the purpose and intent of the business organization to improve society.

## Managing Value Through Stakeholder Management

Stakeholder management is a focal concept in administration and organization narratives (Bandarian, 2008; Kaler, 2003; Shropshire & Hillman, 2007). Key components of any stakeholder value-creating framework are the choices being made; the resources being deployed, including both the tangible and intangible resources (Gilbert & Rasche, 2008; Villalonga, 2004); and the objectives being sought. In any value-creating endeavor, management needs to adequately understand or use the dynamic features of value systems that include feedback systems, time delays, and non-straight cause–effect connections among value system components. Researchers and practitioners generally concur with respect to what drives profits and share prices, that is, long-term cash flow generation (Kothari & Lackner, 2008). In the quest for short-term profits and long-term income, corporate management frequently practices trade-offs to the detriment of their workers. For instance, corporate downsizing and mass layoffs are predicated on revealing better short-term earnings and income and expanding an incentive for all the company's shareholders. On the other hand, numerous effective organizations create value for all their key constituencies by managing to create "win–wins" rather than trade-offs (Salter & Tether, 2006). Put differently, resource utilizing, as opposed to downsizing, is the course these organizations take from their stakeholder point of view (Subramanian &

Youndt, 2005). Concentrating shortsightedly on shareholder value esteem extremely restrains management's understanding of the economics and interdependent nature of stakeholder values which can create a positive and reinforcing loop that can be very robust and advantageous to the firm rather than the vicious cycle of making noncongruent and frequently disparate decision and trade-offs among stakeholder groups.

Porter's value chain model (Porter, 1985) is the best-known model for breaking down how value can be created. This model can assist healthcare managers to achieve a value-creating alignment of decisions, assets, and targets (Hult et al., 2008; Woiceshyn & Falkenberg, 2008). If a business organization can maintain superior value for all stakeholders into the future, it could be able to sustain cash flow into the future (Kaler, 2003; Phillips, Freeman, & Wicks, 2003; Subramanian & Youndt, 2005). Any value-creating activity may rather lead to a value eroding vicious cycle, except if the interests of the considerable stakeholders are congruent. Apart from the shareholders of a healthcare organization, major stakeholders include employees, suppliers, customers, community residents, and governments.

Stakeholders' value long-term vision; for instance, employees crave for a long-term relationship with their employers (organization) for job security, and customer devotion indicates the desire for long-term relationship with a firm. Also, a supplier may be interested in a sustained relationship to secure the customer's patronage, while communities value relationships with businesses that consistently contribute to their welfare. Hence, fruitful businesses include numerous stakeholder value viewpoints in their strategic plan goals. As per the view of Kothari and Lackner's (2006), an organization must bring value to the employees who are behind its productivity, value to the investor who has given capital to it, value to the suppliers who contribute to its market power, value to the consumer who purchases their product and services, and value to the economy or environment in which it operates. The various stakeholders have got independent aims.

Creating long-term stakeholder value is not business as usual activity. Some aspect of the issue lies with the absence of understanding of the features of stakeholder value. Some of these features include interdependency, mixed tangibility, temporality, and commitment intensity. The computation of the social efficiency of the firm is one means to measure stakeholder value. This metric is grounded on the theory that sound relationships and social acceptance between firms and stakeholders are a precondition for sustainable development and economic value creation. In relation to this, healthcare firms should take a more critical look at how they are creating value for their people, communities, and the environment. They should not only be concerned with how they create value for the shareholders alone.

## Sustaining Stakeholder Value

Stakeholder value is creating the best level of return for all stakeholders of an institution, while sustainability is the ability to continue performing an activity indefinitely, having taken into account its impact on natural, social, and human capitals. Sustaining stakeholder value, therefore, is the ability to deliver continuous value to stakeholders over time by taking into consideration the economic, social, and environmental dimensions of its processes and performance. The marketing process, according to Kotler and Armstrong (2010), is tied in with creating value for clients or stakeholders, which consequently creates significant value for stakeholders over the long run. Creating and sustaining stakeholder value is the primary objective of every government. Also, governments connect with a great number of interrelated individuals and constituencies called stakeholders in a network of relationships in creating this value for its publics. These relationships influence the way governments act and their ability to create sustainable stakeholder value.

Stakeholder value is more noticeable in public institutions that seek to create a dialogue with interest groups to achieve policy reform and enhanced service delivery. And stakeholder management is recognized as a central part of an organization's effectiveness in sustaining stakeholder value. According to Ipsos (2009):

> Stakeholders play important roles as advocates, sponsors, partners and agents of change. Much has been written about stakeholder relationships in the private sector and many companies now have dedicated relationship managers and strategies in place to improve and develop external relationships. However, stakeholder management in the public sector still lags some way behind, and is often haphazard. (p. 2)

## Managing Sustainable Stakeholder Value

### *Shaping and Guiding the Stakeholder Dialogue*

From the private sector, it is clear that saving money by cutting back on engaging with your customers and partners is a faulty approach and with this, reputations which are vital, and while hard to win, are easily lost (Ipsos, 2009). Understanding those you work with and those you work for helps to build strong relationships and, ultimately, to achieve your objectives. Research shows that people are more willing to listen to companies with strong reputations, and where there is trust, communication is even more effective (Ipsos, 2009). It is also easy to observe a range of well-known public institutions that have built strong reputations based on clear, cohesive, and identifiable values and cultures (Ipsos, 2009).

Sustainable stakeholder management is about shaping and guiding the stakeholder dialogue to build long-lasting relationships for competitive advantage. Public institutions pursue the objective of sustaining stakeholder value by developing and continuously updating a deep understanding of each stakeholder's present and future needs, and by tailoring the choice, delivery, and communication of their value propositions to these needs as closely as is feasible. They use the information they gather to serve their stakeholders better. The sustainability of stakeholder value flows from understanding of how to deliver what stakeholders need.

The understanding of stakeholder needs is developed by building stakeholder partnerships and not just databases. This means that healthcare institutions must use the data they gather on stakeholders to identify valuable stakeholder actions that will affect value drivers. Capturing the benefits from a stakeholder management approach requires identifying which specific elements drive stakeholder satisfaction through the rigorous targeting of investments.

Successful implementation of sustainable stakeholder value strategy requires fundamental changes in how public institutions think and act, as well as having an understanding of the basic tenets. Public institutions can only sustain stakeholder value by translating their insights into actions. It is a commitment by stakeholders to valuable long-term relationships based on trust and on clear, mutually agreed advantages. The following have been identified as the three elements that champion the course of a successful stakeholder relationship management, which will lead to sustainable value for stakeholders in the long run.

## Demonstrating Good Leadership, Clear Vision, and Focused Direction

It is important that public institutions are well run and are known for their desirable qualities. To achieve this involves having a strong organizational vision and direction, having decision-making ability, and the power of effective implementation. Institutions that rate best among its stakeholders are those with the greatest clarity of purpose. Stakeholders want to be assured that what an organization is doing will add value to them. Just as with customer satisfaction, stakeholder perceptions are greatly influenced by communications which have to be properly nurtured. A healthcare organization that is clear about its objectives and that successfully meets them will be recognized as such by stakeholders.

## Staff Orientation

Good stakeholder relationships are built up over numerous day-to-day interactions. Staff at all levels need to be credible, consistent, and share their organization's objectives. Building a stakeholder relationship is mainly about managing day-to-day working relationships. Thus, the quality of working relationships matters to stakeholders and not just to the effectiveness of management. People make relationships rather than organizations. Perceptions of the quality of a healthcare organization's employees have a strong influence on the value the healthcare organization delivers to its customers and the way that its stakeholders view the healthcare organization. Stakeholders want to deal with experienced and knowledgeable employees of organizations, employees who understand their needs and are able to satisfy them consistently. A strong leadership team is important, but all staff need to realize that they are agents of their organization and represents it. Staff should exhibit consistency in their interactions with stakeholders of the firm. This is because it is the desire of stakeholders to have reliable points of contact with staff who understand their agenda. This entails the development of corporate memory, the ability to direct stakeholders rightly, to staff that can help them best. Where healthcare organizations perform less well, stakeholders are often concerned about the level and experience of the team they are dealing with.

## Excellent Communication

Institutions need to communicate their internal as well as external objectives well and conduct real, two-way conversations with their stakeholders. Institutions build a trustworthy reputation by determining what they want to be known for and being single-minded and united in achieving it. To improve delivery, they need a good understanding of customer needs. A good understanding of what customers want will enable departments to deliver value to stakeholders.

In summary, long-term viability stakeholder value cannot be assured without finding an effective and sustainable social value creation strategy that will address risks and uncertainty issues that emanate from the environment. Thus, while corporations continue to learn from past efforts and seek to develop more sophisticated risk management strategies, the concept of effective and sustainable stakeholder value creation will continue to remain relevant to healthcare organizations. To make delivering a sustainable stakeholder value a "way of life," it must not be seen as a separate project, but as "how we do things." The real challenge is how to create a stakeholder mindset and how to roll it out at a speed that will be sufficiently quick to stay ahead of the pack. Excellent stakeholder management, however, is not something you can simply invoke or turn on or off. Stakeholder management at world-class rates will only come about through persistently pushing the right levers of stakeholder performance.

## Evaluating the Impact of Stakeholder Value Created

There can be multiple actions of a firm that affect a particular stakeholder. The firm may take several such indices into account when making an overall evaluation. In performing a comprehensive assessment of the value derived, stakeholders often must make trade-offs, especially if the value impacts of the actions under consideration are conflicting. Stakeholders may have divergent views on the value created, either because the impacts indeed are different, or because they have been judged differently. By evaluating the impact of stakeholder value, stakeholders can help public institutions to achieve their operational purpose and build trust in the society while solving important problems. Social enterprises play an important role in helping to fulfill societal goals. Porter, Hills, Pfitzer, Patscheke, and Hawkins (2011) in their Harvard article "Measuring Shared Value: How to Unlock Value by Linking Social and Business Results" provides steps for evaluating impact of shareholder's value:

*Step 1:* The starting point for evaluating the impact of stakeholder value created is by identifying the specific social issues that were prioritized to meet a social need. This requires a systematic screening of unmet social needs and gaps with an analysis of how they overlap with the institution's objectives. The authors assert that this step should result in a list of prioritized social issues which a shared value strategy can effectively target.

*Step 2:* After identifying potential social value, the next step is towards the development of a solid business case based on research and analysis on how social improvement can directly affect the value created. This step involves identifying the targets and specifying the activities and costs involved for each shared value opportunity, modelling the potential business and social results relative to the costs, and making a go/no-go decision.

*Step 3:* Track progress against the desired outcome or target, as obtainable in any performance improvement process. This step incorporates tracking inputs and business activities against output performance relative to projections.

*Step 4:* The final step involves the measurement of results and insights gleaned from how to unlock new value. The step focuses on validating the anticipated link between the stakeholder value created (i.e., output or results) and input and determining whether the outlay of corporate resources and efforts produced a good joint return. Insights and lessons from this step will inform opportunities to unlock.

## Conclusion

There are many people and groups involved in providing healthcare. The stakeholders in the healthcare sector were introduced in this chapter. There are healthcare professionals such as doctors and nurses; the parent and customers; government bodies, including the Ministry of Health and the Health Insurance Schemes; and the shareholders (this chapter also differentiates between the shareholder and stakeholders). Stakeholders throughout the healthcare marketing process are crucial because of the success and the continued existence of public health institutions. When stakeholders are satisfied, they reward organizations with resources, provide quality services, and recommend others, but when organizations are unable to deliver, there is the negative word of mouth, complaints, and they can even withdraw their services and terminate their contracts. Acknowledging how important the stakeholders are, this chapter concludes with managing sustainable stakeholder value, which includes using information gathered to service the stakeholders better. The sustainability of stakeholder value flows from understanding how to deliver what stakeholders need. The effective management of the stakeholders is important and valuable toward achieving the strategic goals of the organization.

## Review Questions

1. Briefly explain the stakeholder theory and its importance to healthcare organizations.
2. Differentiate between internal and external stakeholders' needs satisfaction.
3. Explain how stakeholder value can be sustained in healthcare organizations.

## MINI CASE-STUDY: STAKEHOLDERS' VALUE

Elena Specialist hospital, located in Kigali, Rwanda has a 300-bed health facility, with 60 staff which includes five specialists. Dr. Albert, the Chief Medical Director (CMD), of Elena Specialist hospital, upholds the tenet to serve both internal and external customers right. It is one of the best hospitals in town as a result of the fact that the latest medical equipment is available. Elena hospital is known for its quality health service delivery and excellent customer service. The physicians and nurses are well trained and understand their job perfectly well. Elena hospital has been in existence for 18 years and had track records of excellence. The welfare of workers in Elena hospital is of paramount importance because Dr. Albert believes that when an employee is well taken care of; it translates to patients being treated properly, and everyone is happy. Salaries are never late, promotions are never overdue, and other staff welfare packages are put in place.

Patients often noticed Mary, one of the most hardworking and diligent nurses. She has been with Elena Specialist hospital for seven years. She is very calm and patient in carrying out her duties. She is loved by her fellow nurses as well as patients, particularly in-patients. Her words are very soothing to the point that at the sight of her, patients become strengthened even before they are being treated. Mary loves her nursing profession and exhibits a high level of passion in practice. Her hard work and diligence have won her several meritorious service awards at different times; she has also enjoyed promotions to higher levels in her profession. These awards and recognition further encouraged Mary, and she was unrelenting in her duties; she was never proud at any point in time.

Other employees were also relentless in carrying out their duties since it has now become a practice that rewards are given to any deserving staff. This greatly and positively influenced how they go about their job. People within and outside the community visited Elena Specialist hospital with every assurance that their needs will be overly met. They also referred friends and colleagues to the hospital; hence Elena Specialist hospital can boast of a huge customer base.

### Questions
1. Elena Specialist hospital has grown a huge customer base over its years of existence. Do you think effective stakeholder management contributed to the growth? Discuss
2. What do you think could be the fate of Elena hospital in terms of marketing, if Dr. Albert had not prioritized staff welfare?
3. What could be the likely outcome, if the salary structure was very poor and there were delays in payment? How would this outcome affect patients?

# References

Achterkamp, M. C., & Vos, J. F. (2007). Critically identifying stakeholders: evaluating boundary critique as a vehicle for stakeholder identification. Systems Research and Behavioral Science: *The Official Journal of the International Federation for Systems Research, 24*(1), 3–14.

Achterkamp, M. C., & Vos, J. F. J. (2008). Investigating the use of the stakeholder notion in project management literature, a meta-analysis. *International Journal of Project Management, 26*(7), 749–757.

Ananda, J., & Herath, G. (2003). Incorporating stakeholder values into regional forest planning: A value function approach. *Ecological Economics, 45*(1), 75–90.

Aoki, M. (1984). *The co-operative game theory of the firm.* New York, NY: Oxford University Press.

Araujo, L. M., & Bramwell, B. (1999). Stakeholder assessment and collaborative tourism planning: The case of Brazil's Costa Dourada Project. *Journal of Sustainable Tourism, 7*(3/4), 356–378.

Ballejos, L. C., & Montagna, J. M. (2008). Method for stakeholder identification in interorganizational environments. *Requirements Engineering, 13*(4), 281–297.

Bandarian, R. (2008) Exploiting value chain process concepts in research organizations. *International Journal of Value Chain Management, 2*(3), 400–423.

Brickson, S. L. (2005). Organizational identity orientation: Forging a link between organizational identity and organizations' relations with stakeholders. *Administrative Science Quarterly, 50*(4), 576–609.

Brickson, S. L. (2007). Organizational identity orientation: The genesis of the role of the firm and distinct forms of social value. *Academy of Management Review, 32*(3), 864–888.

Bryson, J. M. (2004). What to do when stakeholders matter: Stakeholder identification and analysis techniques. *Public Management Review, 6*(1), 21–53.

Bundy, J., Shropshire, C., & Buchholtz, A. K. (2013). Strategic cognition and issue salience: Toward an explanation of firm responsiveness to stakeholder concerns. *Academy of Management Review, 38*(3), 352–376.

Corbin, C. L., Kelley, S. W., & Schwartz, R. W. (2001). Concepts in service marketing for healthcare professionals. *The American Journal of Surgery, 181*(1), 1–7.

Department for International Development, UK. (2002). *Tools for development: A handbook for those engaged in development activity.* Retrieved from http://www.unssc.org/web1/ls/downloads/toolsfordevelopment%20dfid.pdf

Donaldson, T., & Preston, L. E. (1995). The stakeholder theory of the corporation: Concepts, evidence, and implications. *Academic Management Review, 20*(1), 65–91.

English Nature. (2002). *Revealing the value of nature.* Peterborough, England: Author.

Fontaine, C., Haarman, A., & Schmid, S. (2006). The stakeholder theory. *Edlays Education, 1*, 1–33.

Freeman, R. E. (1984). *Strategic management: A stakeholder approach.* Boston, MA: Pitman.

Freeman, R. E. (2004). The stakeholder approach revisited. *Zeitschrift für Wirtschafts-und Unternehmensethik, 5*(3), 228–254.

Freeman, R. E. (2010). *Strategic management: A stakeholder approach.* Cambridge, MA: Cambridge University Press.

Freeman, R. E., Wicks, A. C., & Parmar, B. (2004). Stakeholder theory and "the corporate objective revisited." *Organization Science, 15*(3), 364–369.

Friedman, A. L., & Miles, S. (2006). *Stakeholders: Theory and practice.* New York, NY: Oxford University Press on Demand.

Gilbert, D. U., & Rasche, A. (2008). Opportunities and problems of standardized ethics initiatives–a stakeholder theory perspective. *Journal of Business Ethics, 82*(3), 755–773.

Hair, J. F., Bush, R. P., & Ortinau, D. J. (2000). *Marketing research: A practical approach for the new millennium.* Boston, MA: McGraw-Hill.

Huhmann, B. A., & Limbu, Y. B. (2016). Content and compliance of pharmaceutical social media marketing. *Marketing Intelligence & Planning, 34*(7), 977–999.

Hult, G. T. M., Ketchen, D. J., Griffith, D. A., Chabowski, B. R., Hamman, M. K., Dykes, B. J., & Cavusgil, S. T. (2008). An assessment of the measurement of performance in international business research. *Journal of International Business Studies, 39*(6), 1064–1080.

Ipsos MORI. (2009). Understanding your stakeholders. A best practice guide for the public sector. *Social Research Institute.* Retrieved from https://www.ipsos.com/sites/default/files/publication/1970-01/sri-understanding-stakeholders-november-2009.pdf

Jennings, S. F., & Lockie, S. (2002). *Democratisation and capacity building in coastal zone decision-making in Australia: The application of stakeholder analysis and social mapping.* Paper presented at the Coastal Zone Asia Pacific Conference, Bangkok, TH.

Kaler, J. (2003). Differentiating stakeholder theories. *Journal of Business Ethics, 46*(1), 71–83.

Kothari, A., & Lackner, J. (2006). A value based approach to management. *Journal of Business & Industrial Marketing, 21*(4), 243–249.

Kotler, P., & Armstrong, G. (2010). *Principles of marketing.* White Plains, NY: Pearson Education.

Limbu, Y. B., McKinley, C., & Temperini, V. (2019). A longitudinal examination of FDA warning and untitled letters issued to pharmaceutical companies for violations in drug promotion standards. *Journal of Consumer Affairs, 53*(1), 3–23.

Mathur, V. N., Price, A. D., Austin, S. A., & Moobela, C. (2007). *Defining, identifying and mapping stakeholders in the assessment of urban sustainability.* Loughborough, England: Loughborough University.

Mitchell, R. K., Agle, B. R., & Wood, D. J. (1997). Toward a theory of stakeholder identification and salience: Defining the principle of who and what really counts. *Academy of Management Review, 22*(4), 853–886.

Moore, M. H. (1995). *Creating public value: Strategic management in government.* Cambridge, MA: Harvard University Press.

Phillips, R., Freeman, R. E., & Wicks, A. C. (2003). What stakeholder theory is not. *Business Ethics Quarterly, 13*(4), 479–502.

Porter, M. E. (1985). Competitive advantage: Creating and sustaining superior performance. New York, NY: FreePress.

Porter, M. E., Hills, G., Pfitzer, M., Patscheke, S., & Hawkins, E. (2011). Measuring shared value: How to unlock value by linking social and business results. *Harvard Business School.* https://www.hbs.edu/faculty/Publication%20Files/Measuring_Shared_Value_57032487-9e5c-46a1-9bd8-90bd7f1f9cef.pdf

Rainey, H. G. (1999). Using comparisons of public and private organizations to assess innovative attitudes among members of organizations. *Public Productivity & Management Review,* 130–149.

Rawlins, B. (2006). *Prioritizing stakeholders for public relations.* Salt Lake City, UT: Institute for Public Relations.

Salter, A., & Tether, B. S. (2006, April 7). Innovation in services through the looking glass of innovation studies. Background paper for Advanced Institute of Management (AIM) Research's Grand Challenge on Service Science. Retrieved from http://citeseerx.ist.psu.edu/viewdoc/download?doi=10.1.1.103.7928&rep=rep1&type=pdf

Savage, G. T., Nix, T. W., Whitehead, C. J., & Blair, J. D. (1991). Strategies for assessing and managing organizational stakeholders. *Academy of Management Perspectives, 5*(2), 61–75.

Scott, S. G., & Lane, V. R. (2000). A stakeholder approach to organizational identity. *Academy of Management Review, 25*(1), 43–62.

Shropshire, C., & Hillman, A. J. (2007). A longitudinal study of significant change in stakeholder management. *Business & Society, 46*(1), 63–87.

Subramanian, M., & Youndt, M. A. (2005). The influence of intellectual capital on the types of innovative capabilities. *Academy of Management Journal, 48*(3), 450–463.

Thomas, R. K. (2004). *Marketing health services. The evolving societal and healthcare context.* Chicago, IL: Health Administration Press.

Thomas, R. K. (2008). *Health services marketing: A practitioner's guide.* New York, NY: Springer Science & Business Media.

Villalonga, B. (2004). Intangible resources, Tobin'sq, and sustainability of performance differences. *Journal of Economic Behavior & Organization, 54*(2), 205–230.

Woiceshyn, J., & Falkenberg, L. (2008). Value creation in knowledge-based firms: Aligning problems and resources. *Academy of Management Perspectives, 22*(2), 85–99.

# 8

## *Consumer Behavior in Healthcare Service Encounters*

### Chapter Outline

- Introduction
- Consumers' Interactions With Healthcare Service Operators
- The Multiple Steps in the Healthcare Service Purchase Process
- Healthcare Service Customers' Needs and Expectations in Relation to Service Offerings
- Disconfirmation Theory
- Customer Expectation in Products and Services
- Monitoring Customer Needs and Expectations Constantly
- Customer Expectation in Healthcare Services
- Expectation of the Aged in Healthcare Services
- Service Evaluation by Healthcare Service Customers
- Cues and Signals of Service Quality
- The Healthcare Service Business as a System
- Conclusion
- Review Questions
- Mini Case Study With Discussion Questions
- References

*Marketing in Healthcare-Related Industries*, pages 173–204
Copyright © 2020 by Information Age Publishing
All rights of reproduction in any form reserved.

## Chapter Outcome

By the end of this chapter, the reader will be able to

- define consumer behavior,
- discuss how customers interact with healthcare service operations,
- illustrate the multiple steps in the purchase process for healthcare services,
- discuss customers' needs and expectations in relation to healthcare services offerings,
- explain how customers may find it difficult to evaluate healthcare services, and
- discuss the healthcare service business as a system.

## Introduction

Consumer behavior is defined as the behavior that consumers show in searching for, purchasing, using, evaluating, and disposing of products and services which they believe will satisfy their needs (Schiffman & Kanuk, 2007). A health service encounter could be defined as a period of time during which a customer directly interacts with a service (Shostack, 1985). According to Bitner (1990), health service encounters also pertain to the "discrete, separate, and distinct events and behavior, as well as a customer's interaction with all the dimensions of a health service, such as the physical surroundings and the health service contact employees" (p. 72). Crosby, Evans, and Cowles (1990) also argue that a health service encounter occurs whenever the patient interacts with a frontline healthcare employee, and the healthcare employee's behavior affects the patient's perception of the service quality.

## Consumers' Interactions With Healthcare Service Operators

One issue that affects a patient's interaction with healthcare service operations is sometimes the age of the individual delivering the service. Sometimes an older doctor is perceived as more knowledgeable and experienced than a doctor with youthful looks. Although customer consumption behavior is mainly influenced by social and psychographic factors like family size, income, and self-image (Alalaakkola, 1996), the age of the individual rendering the services is seen to impact a customer's consumption pattern. What sometimes compounds this issue in a health service encounter is the increase in the consumption of healthcare services among older consumers

(50+; Alalaakkola, 1996). The two main questions that arise as a result of this is whether elderly customers (people above 50 years) would opt for elderly customer-contact individuals or whether relatively mature customers (people between 35–49 years) customers prefer relatively mature customer-contact individuals?

As the production and the consumption of services are simultaneous, customer contact persons should be in the best position to adapt the healthcare service rendered to achieve what the customer desires, explicitly from the service encounter (Parasuraman, Zeithaml, & Berry, 1985). The adaptation of services to suit customers will consider what and/or how services are delivered. These adaptations can be perceived as having two dimensions: first, the ability to modify the service rendered and second, the ability to accept other behaviors (Bettencourt & Gwinner, 1996; Gwinner, Bitner, Brown, & Kumar, 2005). In the first dimension, the tailoring of or uniquely created service offering to meet the expectations of individual customers is referred to as the adaptation for service. In the second dimension, the interactive behavior exhibited concerning the wishes or needs of individual customers, such as vocabulary or gestures is also referred to as the adaptation of interpersonal behavior (Weitz, Sunjan, & Sunjan,1986). In the hospital, during patient interaction, for instance, a doctor might get the best out of a patient by speaking a local language rather than insisting on communicating in English, French, or other national official language.

Customer-contact persons in health service delivery should be able to comprehend what customer limitations and predispositions are, if they have the ability to explain events in a service interaction and adequately adapt their behavior (1986). This way, more successful health outcomes might be reached. For a customer-contact person to be able to acquire this skill, much will depend on the behavioral traits of the customer-contact individual, and the drive of the customer-contact individual to deliver service excellence (Sujan, Weitz, & Kumar, 1994).

Customers will have the tendency to associate themselves with individuals whom they share similar features and backgrounds with. This is termed as the theory of person perception and is explained by Newcomb (1956) as the similarity/attraction hypothesis. The similarity/attraction hypothesis argues that people are attracted to others with whom they perceive to share similar characteristics, and in a service management setting, this may appear as a consumer's preference for a customer-contact person with shared characteristics (Churchill, Collins, & Strang, 1975; Gadel, 1964; Mills, Chase, & Marguiles, 1983).

The issue of the age of the contact employee and the type of service being rendered play a role in determining how customers interact with service operations. A study conducted by Kang and Hillery on the role of an elderly person and a fairly mature salesperson serving the elderly or the fairly mature customers within a retail-clothing setting, found that elderly customers had more favorable attitudes towards elderly salespersons in general and fairly mature customers preferred elderly salespersons. This, in summary, could be as a result of the fact that the elderly exhibit more concern and more easily give necessary details, which explains the preference of both elderly and fairly mature customers (1998). Apart from the study conducted by Kang and Hillery (1998), Wägar and Lindqvist (2010) also espoused that "age of the customer-contact person might vary with services that differ in their levels of search qualities, experience qualities and credence qualities" (p. 514). This outcome of age could change, for example, with respect to retailing of technical appliances and clothing, which are high in search qualities, lower on experience and credence qualities; or barbering and hairdressing services, which are high in experience qualities, lower on search and credence qualities (Wägar & Lindqvist, 2010).

Another issue to be considered under how customers interact with service operations will be the role of emotional satisfaction in service encounters. A central element in service quality management is the role of emotion, as it determines the response customers will be given in their service encounter, as asserted by Oliver, Rust, and Varki (1997). Customer evaluations of service encounters are connected with the behaviors of the frontline service employees (Hartline, Maxham, & McKee, 2000). However, there are no clear models in the literature in this research area (Grönroos, 2001). Liljander and Strandvik (1995) assert that customers will have a strong relationship with and be more committed to the organization if they develop a positive emotional response towards individual contact employees. The set of emotional responses explicitly elicited during consumption experiences is the concept of consumption emotion according to the satisfaction literature (Westbrook & Oliver, 1991). From prior research, one responds to events in certain ways to maintain positive emotions, like happiness, and to avoid negative emotions, like depression (Stauss & Neuhaus, 1997). Wong (2004), revealed through a study on Australian retail customers that emotional satisfaction and service quality are positively associated with each other and also with customer loyalty and relationship quality. The article further stated that the best predictor of customer loyalty has to do with the customers' feelings of loyalty while the best predictor of relationship quality deals with the feeling of happiness.

Additionally, an article titled, "The Effect of Gaze on Consumers' Encounter Evaluation" written by Andersson, Wastlaund, and Kristensson (2016) confirms the favorable effects of receiving direct eye contact with an employee during a service encounter. From the study, participants who received a direct gaze reportedly felt more affirmed, and their social impression of the frontline employee was more positive, as compared with that of participants who received an averted gaze. Moreover, the participants who received a direct gaze also reported more satisfaction with the encounter, thereby, indicating additional positive short-term effects. However, the study also showed that the purchase situation could moderate the effect of gaze, and a gaze can produce an opposite effect. When a consumer is buying an embarrassing product, a direct gaze generates more negative emotions and lower levels of encounter satisfaction. Past research by Wirth, Sacco, Hugenberg, and Williams (2010) demonstrated that gaze is a powerful regulator of ongoing social interactions, and their results suggest that the effect of a gaze starts early in the social interaction. In their study, the participants reached their assessment of satisfaction before they received a verbal response from the frontline employee, which tends to support the importance of employee-displayed eye contact. However, their research also shows that the specific purchase situation is an important moderator of this relationship and the positive effect between direct gaze and encounter satisfaction, is not valid when the purchase situation involves feelings of embarrassment. This goes to show how customers' interactions with service operations relate to the emotions of the customer and the perception of the customer with regards to the service operations.

## The Multiple Steps in the Healthcare Service Purchase Process

According to the stage model of the purchase process for services, consumers of services go through three major stages including the prepurchase stage, the service encounter stage, and the post-encounter stage (Lovelock & Wirtz, 2011; Tsiotsou & Wirtz, 2012), see Figure 8.1 on the stage model of the purchase process for services.

### Pre-Purchase Stage

In this first stage, the customer's need triggers a search for information and an evaluation of alternatives before they make a purchase decision. Furthermore, the processes involved in arriving at a decision for a service as compared to that of a product/good is more complex due to the nature of services (Fisk, 1981). A consumer's expertise, knowledge, and perceived risk play essential roles in this pre-purchase stage. Triggering needs can occur in a number of ways such as the oblivious mind, which is responsible for

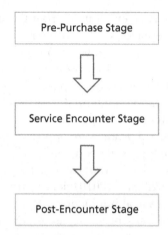

**Figure 8.1** The stage model of the purchase process for services. *Source:* Lovelock & Wirtz, 2011.

impulse purchases; internal conditions, such as the desire for food; and external sources, such as the marketing mix, to name a few (Tsiotsou & Wirtz, 2012). Conversely, consumers can first recognize a need or problem and be motivated to search for a solution to satisfy them in what is called planned-purchase behavior. Figure 8.2 shows the pre-purchase stage process.

---

## The Service Encounter Stage

This is the second stage of the purchase process, where experiences and value are cocreated by consumers and providers of the service while evaluating the service experience (Tsiotsou & Wirtz, 2012). Bowden (2009) asserts that engagement is applicable to services because of the existence of an interaction between the consumers and the frontline employees in the service process, and this creates a reciprocal relationship. Consumer engagement is the emotional tie that binds the consumer to the service provider as feelings of confidence, integrity, pride, and passion in a firm/ brand are part of the interaction (Goldsmith, 2012; McEwen, 2004). Therefore, the motivation, the ability, and the knowledge to provide and integrate various resources are necessary for customers to become engaged in the coproduction of a service or in cocreation of value during the service encounter stage (Schneider & Bowen,1995; Lusch & Vargo, 2006). Involving a sequence of related events in the service encounter is generally considered a service delivery process occurring at different points in time. This supports the assertion that consumers enter a *service factory* when they visit a service delivery entity (Noone & Mattila, 2009).

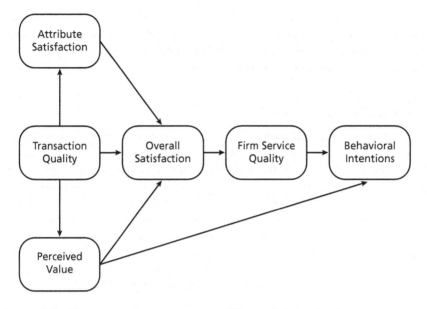

**Figure 8.2**   The pre-purchase stage. *Source:* Tsiotsou & Wirtz, 2012.

The proposed service encounter model is an integration of the *servuction* model which combines the terms, *service* and *production* and the servicescape/environmental model. The servuction system contains a technical core which is invisible to the customer, and the service delivery system that is visible to and experienced by the consumer (Eiglier & Langeard, 1977; Langeard, Bateson, Lovelock, & Eiglier, 1981). According to Tsiotsou and Wirtz (2012, pp. 156–157), the servuction system includes all the interactions that together make up a typical consumer experience in a high-contact service. The system suggests that consumers interact with the service environment, service employees and even other consumers present during the service encounter. Service environments or servicescapes, as cited by Bitner (1992), refer to the style and appearance of the physical surroundings and other experiential elements consumers at a service firm encounter during service delivery. The four purposes of servicescapes, as stated by Lovelock and Wirtz (2011), are to engineer the consumer experience and shape consumer behavior, convey the planned image of the firm and support its positioning and differentiation strategy, serve as part of the value proposition, facilitate the service encounter, and enhance both service quality and productivity.

Lovelock and Wirtz (2011) highlight that in the service context, low-contact entails little physical contact between service providers and consumers. This low-contact could also occur at arm's length via electronic or physical distribution channels. The authors add that many high-contact and medium-contact services are becoming low-contact services due to consumers' increasing desire for convenience.

---

### *The Post-Encounter Stage*

In service consumption, the last stage is the post-encounter stage, which involves how individuals or consumers respond to the service being rendered (Tsiotsou & Wirtz, 2012). When performance perceptions of individual consumers are within the expectation range, such individuals are likely to make repeat purchases, remain loyal to the service provider, and ultimately spread positive word-of-mouth. According to Oliver, Rust, and Varki (1997), consumers that experience service performance exceeding the expected level exhibit consumer delight. This is exhibited in the form of an unexpected increase in performance levels and of surprise and excitement triggered by arousal and pleasure, or of joy and happiness as a result of a positive effect. Customer delight might not always act in favor of the health service firm, because it raises consumers' expectation and can lead to consumers becoming dissatisfied if service levels return to the previously lower levels. Consequently, it will probably take more effort to satisfy/delight them in the future. Figure 8.3 shows the post-encounter stage process.

---

## Health Service Customers' Needs and Expectations in Relation to Service Offerings

The satisfaction of customers and/or the overall service quality is a crucial determinant in the comparison between what the customer expects of the service rendered and the perception of the actual service received (Solomon, Surprenant, Czepiel, & Gutman, 1985; Walker, 1995; Zeithaml, Berry, & Parasuraman, 1993). From a broader perspective, expectation, as used in the organizational literature, is seen first from the angle where it focuses on the behavior. This behavior is explained in relation to the subjective probability that if a particular outcome is expected, it will be as a result of a given behavior (Bardwell, 1984; Landy & Trumbo, 1980). As noted by Tsiotsou and Wirtz (2012), "more broadly, expectations reflect an individual's subjective probabilities about the current or future existence of a particular state of affairs" (p. 55).

Zeithaml et al. (1993) and Boulding, Kalna, Staelin, and Zeithaml (1993) threw more light on the issues relating to the definition by highlighting two

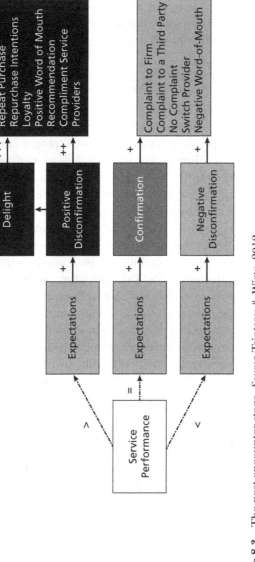

**Figure 8.3** The post-encounter stage. *Source* Tsiotsou & Wirtz, 2012.

principal conceptualizations of expectations. In the opinion of these authors, there was a clear difference between prediction made by customers about what was going to happen during an impending transaction or exchange and the prediction by service providers. The authors then concluded by stating that the expectations of customers are not the same as the ideal or desired standards of those customers. Zeithaml et al. (1993) further emphasized their argument by stating an example, where a customer perceived an expensive restaurant to have fine wines available in stock even though the said customer might not be interested in purchasing any.

### Customer Needs and Expectations

The expectations of customers have a direct link with the complaints resulting from the post-purchase effect (Santos & Boote, 2003). These post-purchase effects, depending on the individual, ranges from delight, satisfaction, and dissatisfaction. These affective behaviors depicted as a result of satisfaction and delight are termed as compliments (Santos & Boote, 2003). Alternatively, behaviors as a result of dissatisfaction are termed as complaints, which increases in its strength as more dissatisfaction is experienced. As Gilbert, Lumpkin, and Dant (1992) explained, people create a yardstick for themselves through their expectations in their quest to evaluate the attractiveness and desirability of outcomes, events, people, products, and services, among others. Although primary care physicians may refer patients to use more specialized care, ultimately, the patients make the final decision of the need for healthcare. Since customer expectations have grown rapidly over the past 3 decades, the success of healthcare providers is dependent on their ability to meet consumers' growing needs and expectations (Vogenberg & Santilli, 2018). As healthcare continues to move toward a patient-centered approach, it is important that healthcare providers shift their focus on consumers' needs rather than their own needs.

### Forming Expectations

Communication directed at the market, the characteristics of the individual, how the individual communicates to others, or the necessities of the individual are the basis upon which expectations can be based (Leventhal, 2008). "Additionally, customer pre-attitudes or even the traditional marketing mix can influence what the consumer will expect from a product or service" (2008, p. 51). A consumer's expectation can be formed on the basis of a previous encounter with a particular institution and its structural attributes. *Predictive* or *will expectations* are those that the consumer thinks will happen in the next service encounter, while *should expectations* are those that the consumer thinks should happen in the next encounter" (2008, p. 51). Consumer prospects can take the form of generally acceptable ranges or individualistic perceptions contrary to the general practice in connection to the marketplace or the lessons learnt by the individual, as he or she interacted with the specific product or service in the past (Leventhal, 2008).

The needs of customers and, thus, their expectations, can be divided into three categories; namely, the *must needs*, which the customer does not think about expressing, but will miss if not provided for or the *expected needs*, which are those that customers are able to articulate when asked about what they want; or they could be exciting requirements which are those *unexpected needs* that produce great satisfaction. The must needs impose a duty on the providers of the goods and services to continuously enhance their products or services. When consumers of a specific group of products or services maintain their product or service providers as a result of having their needs met and find little reason to move to alternate providers, this is called the adaptation theory (Gilbert et al., 1992). This behavior, however, changes as customers experience a transformation in expectation and now begin to consider the best options to take as to whether to stay with the current provider or move to other providers.

## Disconfirmation Theory

Disconfirmation or confirmation theory traces its roots to the adaptation theory, which was as a result of Helson's (1964) works. On a basic level, it is defined as whether or not the service delivery or the product was able to meet the expectations of the consumer. More specifically, if the consumer's expectation is met, it is classified as confirmed expectation, and in events where the expectation is not met, it is classified as disconfirmed expectations. The theory, as a standards model, rests on the fact contrary to when service performance was equal to predicted expectations. It was said that a consumer was indifferent, under this model, when performance was equal to desired expectations; satisfaction is said to be exceedingly higher. A critical analysis of the disconfirmation expectation literature suggests that the theory only provides a partial understanding of the satisfaction causes. It is, therefore, worth noting that in response to the lack of acknowledgement of the desired expectations as a source of customer satisfaction, a model was formulated based on disconfirmation of expectations theory which regards delight as an affective state in addition to satisfaction. Positive disconfirmation occurs when consumers are satisfied, and ideal expectations are met. This is the level where delight and satisfaction occur leading to complimentary behavior.

To summarize, customer requirements were established as the basis of the emotional conditions like a consumer being pleased or a consumer being unhappy or upset with the product offering or service offering, thus, compelling the consumer to compliment or complain about the providers of the offerings rendered or the offerings themselves. Further, the types of customer requirements were identified and compiled. These requirements took the form of customer needs with three categories of needs identified. Lastly, the theory based on the consumer's ability to adjust and disassociate with a given situation was noted as the dominant model for comprehending customer requirements and how unsatisfied needs could drive customers to portray behaviors that exhibited their distaste for the product or service rendered. Management would, therefore, be in a better position to put measures in place that would reduce the occurrence of the distress encountered by their customers.

## Customer Expectation in Products and Services

The quality of a product can be easily recognized by visible factors such as style, hardness, color, label, feel, package, fit, and functionality. Product quality is determined by the number of occurrences relating to its internal and external failures (Garvin, 1983 as cited in Parasuraman et al., 1985). The intangible nature of a service, coupled with the heterogeneous nature of the service in relation to providers in the same service industry and instances where the creators of the service deliver it themselves, has made the determination of its quality very difficult. Table 8.1 shows customer expectations and likely outcomes.

**TABLE 8.1 Customer Expectations and Outcomes**

| Expectation | Dis/Confirmation | Affective State | Outcome |
|---|---|---|---|
| Ideal | Positive Disconfirmation | Delight | Compliments |
| Should Be | | | |
| Desired | | Satisfaction | |
| Predicted | Confirmation | Indifference | |
| Minimum Tolerable | Negative Disconfirmation | Acceptance | |
| Intolerable | | Dissatisfaction | Complaints |
| Worst Imaginable | | | |

*Source:* Parasuraman et al., 1985

Ultimately, there are different products produced and consumed at the same time in health service delivery. In health services, as customers compare their expectations to the actual performance rendered, the quality of the service is being judged. Customers seek consistent performance delivery and service satisfaction, which is determined by whether there was positive or negative disconfirmation of expectations (Parasuraman et al., 1985). Additionally, the outcome of a service and the process involved in delivery are vital in the provision of the service. Sasser, Olsen, and Wyckoff (1978), as cited by Parasuraman et al. (1985), assert that service quality is determined by three factors, namely: the items for production, the means of production, and the manpower involved in the process.

Grönroos (1982) as cited by Parasuraman et al. (1985) has defined two types of quality: the technical (outcomes) and the functional (delivery). Additionally, Lehtinen (1982), as cited by Parasuraman et al. (1985), identifies three service quality dimensions; namely, the *corporate quality* (image), the *physical quality*, and the *interactive quality*. In relation to other service qualities, expectations have been identified in the literature, including reliability, responsiveness, competence, access and approachability, courtesy, communication, credibility, security, understanding customers, and finally the tangible aspects of service delivery (Parasuraman et al., 1985). The intangible nature of the service, together with the processes involved in the service being rendered, helps in understanding the complexities associated with the varying nature of services (Lim, Tang, & Jackson, 1999).

According to Kano, Seraku, Takahashi, and Tsuji's (1984), in the theory of attractive quality, customer needs can be separated into the three following categories:

1. *Must-be requirements:* These are needs that satisfy a minimum acceptable service level. Although they are implicit, obvious, and unspoken, they should not be neglected, but rather guaranteed and monitored by the service organization because their fulfilment will increase satisfaction.
2. *One-dimensional requirements:* These are needs expected by customers who usually explicitly demand these of the service organization.
3. *Attractive requirements:* These are latent needs, that is, they are not expected by customers because customers themselves are not conscious of them. Normally, customers do not think, or do not know, that fulfilling these needs could be helpful to them. Even if these needs are not met, this will not result in dissatisfaction (Coye, 2004). Their fulfilment creates satisfaction or delight (Berman, 2005; Kim & Mattila, 2013).

In service quality research, expectations are defined as the desires or wants of customers, that is, what service providers should offer rather than would offer (Parasuraman, Zeithaml, & Berry, 1988). In other terms, needs differ from expectations because needs are thought to underlie expectations (Chiu & Lin, 2004) residing more rooted in the psyche and tending to be more unconscious and global in contrast to expectations, which are more conscious, accessible, and specific in nature (Schneider & Bowen, 1995).

The needs hierarchy theory, as conceptualized by Maslow (1970), rank the basic human needs in the order of importance. Aigbavboa (2016) asserts that the needs depicted by Maslow arrange themselves in order of prepotency. He further stated that the appearance of a new need shows that the previous need has been satisfied, showing that "no need or drive can be treated as if it were isolated or discrete; thus, every drive is related to the state of satisfaction or dissatisfaction of other drives" (Aigbavboa, 2016, p. 11). Maslow believes that certain behavior is motivated by a need and will cease once the need is satisfied; however, as needs are satisfied, new needs will come to the fore (1970). Therefore, the hierarchy of needs is created and cover physiological needs, safety needs, need to belong and love needs, esteem needs, and need for self-actualization. Needs are satisfied in order, according to how they rank in importance, starting with the most basic needs and progressively growing more complex. Maslow (1970), hence, indicates that the need to fulfill higher-order needs such as influence and personal development only arises when lower order needs of physical and emotional well-being are satisfied. Conversely, if lower needs cannot be met, higher needs will not be pursued for satisfaction (Aigbavboa, 2016). The hierarchy of needs has been applied to the business and management industry to help managers understand employee motivation.

Satisfaction is closely related to expectations. Studies on satisfaction using disconfirmation of expectations propose that satisfaction is the result of a comparison of what was expected and that which was received (Woodruff, Cadotte, & Jenkins, 1983). Erevelles and Leavitt (1992) mention that post-purchase evaluation of a product can be explained, at least in part, by a comparison of the prepurchase performance. Also, Spreng, MacKenzie, and Olshavsky (1996) stretch the disconfirmation of expectations theory to include desires by developing a new model which integrates desires and expectations. Tse and Wilton (1988) suggest that in addition to the influences from expected performance and subjective disconfirmation, perceived performance exerts direct influence on satisfaction. Hence, the expectancy disconfirmation model claims that the user's satisfaction results from the response to the close connection between an individual's expectations and the actual performance of a product (Oliver, 1980). In relation to the public housing subsidy scheme, satisfaction is regarded as a function of the interrelationship between what beneficiaries expect from the government and their perceptions of the house they have received. That is, the quality of the houses received, and the satisfaction derived from the housing services provided (Aigbavboa, 2016).

According to Reisig and Chandek (2001), the expectancy theory is divided into a four-stage process. In the first stage, consumers will develop expectations of a product and product performance, based on their product knowledge or other normative factors (Tse & Wilton, 1988; Oliver, 1980; Woodruff et al., 1983). In the second and third stages, they form certain perceptions about the performance of that product. This perception of the product's performance is then compared to the initial expectations of the individual (Aigbavboa, 2016). In the final stage, a consumer compares their expectations of the product to their experience with the product (Aigbavboa, 2016). According to Oliver (1980), the degree to which perceptions of performance match expectations determines the type of disconfirmation a consumer experiences. When a consumer's expectations are exceeded, positive disconfirmation occurs, likely leading to satisfaction. When expectations are met, zero disconfirmation occurs, having no effect on satisfaction, and when expectations are neither met nor exceeded, negative disconfirmation occurs, leading to dissatisfaction (2016). Reisig and Chandek (2001) and Aigbavboa (2016) have found that satisfaction is not only affected by disconfirmation, but also by expectations and performance. Performance is positively related to user satisfaction, where an increase in a firm's performance leads to an increase in user satisfaction. Oppositely, user satisfaction is inversely related to expectations, where the lower the expectations, the higher the satisfaction (Aigbanboa, 2016).

## Monitoring Customer Needs and Expectations Constantly

As attractive health brands live and die by the will of market consumers, companies must constantly collect information about consumers' behavior as well as their culture. This helps build a better brand aimed at satisfying consumer needs and meeting consumer expectations. For example, the iPhone® was the most attractive smartphone on the market during the period in which Apple® introduced it. Subsequently, a large number of consumers switched from using phone brands like Nokia®, Sony Ericsson®, Motorola®, and other similar brands to using the iPhone. In later years, Samsung® understood consumer tastes and needs. As such, Samsung was able to launch the Galaxy® brand which was more appealing to consumers. Samsung used features and big screens to differentiate the strategy of the Galaxy Brand. The company also used a successful marketing strategy through which it offered different options of brand new smartphones, targeting different consumers, including low-end smartphones for the developing world. The study demonstrates that research on brand switching should continue to be investigated across different industries, to include the influence of various factors on consumer behavior toward replacing a brand. Even though many managers claim they have the knowledge of how to make their brands attractive, in reality, they must conduct frequent market research analyses to learn from competitors and consumers. It is important that managers should not rely on their existing knowledge to predict how to make an attractive brand, as research has shown that consumers and suppliers have different perceptions of the determinants of brand switching. To determine the attractiveness of a brand would require putting in place appropriate strategies to prevent the market share from eroding.

Al-Kwifi and Ahmed (2015) propose a continuing exploration of the influence of online technology, such as social networks and discussion boards to monitor how consumers describe and discuss their personal experience with a brand. In doing so, a brand can learn how consumers utilize their product daily, how it adds value, what they like and dislike about the brand, and what features they would like to see in future products. Such information represents an excellent source of new ideas to improve the brand value as well as to discover the reasons why competitor brands might be more attractive to consumers. This interactive tracking system has proved to be highly efficient for certain industries, such as the hotel and tourism sectors, in which users are asked to provide feedback.

Many companies are tracking this information about their own and competitors' brands to enable them to develop strategies that improve their brand image in the market. These tracking systems are a good source of information about consumers' interest in and ideas about most products and services. For high technology products, however, where the rate of technological change is high and technology standards are difficult to determine, defining consumers' optimum preferences is a challenging task, because preferences constantly change while each product represents a unique feature that might achieve different objectives. Therefore, selecting the optimal preferences for products requires collecting information from multiple sources and defining the most critical product features that would make the brand attractive to consumers. Given that brand switching behavior is a dynamic and complex process, it is important that future research explores this issue from diverse perspectives and introduces new approaches to interpret this behavior.

## Customer Expectation in Healthcare Services

Patients' expectations in healthcare continue to increase and thus, not meeting their expectations can lead to dissatisfaction with the service. Healthcare firms must understand and use marketing and consumer behavior strategies if they want to meet the increasing demands of patient expectations. The major changes undergone by the health services can be attributed to external factors like a rise in other providers of that particular service (Gilbert et al., 1992). This, therefore, makes it essential for providers in the health sector to understand the customers' expectations and requirements, thus, giving providers in the health sector the ability to compete effectively and maintain their customers. A basic expectation among hospital patients in developing countries is the assurance that they will be attended to by skilled and competent staff who will treat them professionally and efficiently, and perform procedures correctly (Andaleeb, 2001). Workers or professionals in the health sector are equipped with specific skills such as competence, which include skillful and timely medical care and medication administration, as well as the experience of the health professional.

The care given to individuals by health professionals can be categorized into professional attributes such as the abilities of the providers, surgical skills of doctors, and accuracy in diagnosing conditions, as well as behavioral attributes such as the ability to establish good relationships with patients. The behavioral attributes of health professionals are communicated through eye contact, attitude, and ability and are especially important in matters of patient care, approaching sensitive subjects and questions with caution, and protecting confidential patient data.

## Expectation of the Aged in Healthcare Services

Apart from the treatment given to patients with regards to healthcare, special attention is needed in services delivered to the aged. Older patients with chronic conditions have high outcome expectations. Since the aging population is growing, largely due to rising life expectancy, extra attention should be given to them due to their weaker conditions and inability to advocate for themselves. Issues concerning the aged and their health often involve external/third party decision-makers who are responsible for determining the aged person's needs pertaining to safety, emotional support, and other crucial matters. This often burdens these decision-makers as they will have to leave their elderly family member elsewhere and, in most cases, permanently. In the process of delivery of service to the aged, services must be of the highest quality, the operating environment must be superior, and the decision-makers involved must be committed to seeking the best interest of the aged above all else.

## Service Evaluation by Healthcare Service Customers

Customers have different criteria or starting posts for their evaluating services rendered to them. Although the customer's contact with a healthcare employee plays a significant role in how customers perceive the service, there are many factors that can affect and even present obstacles for customer evaluation.

### The Role of the Emotional State of the Customer

A central element in service quality management that is gaining much attention is the role of the emotional state of the customer (Oliver, 1997); however, there are no clear models available in this research area in the literature (Grönroos, 2001). Emotion, as seen from literature, is a fundamental attribute in satisfaction, and it is proposed that customer satisfaction should include a separate emotional component (Cronin, Brady, & Hult, 2000). Indeed, Stauss and Neuhaus (1997) contend that past research on satisfaction has focused largely on the cognitive component of emotion, but the affective component has received little attention. Further, it was argued by Liljander and Strandvik (1997) that customer satisfaction includes both affective, thus, emotional and cognitive components. According to the satisfaction literature, the set of emotional responses elicited specifically during consumption experiences is the concept of consumption emotion, as asserted by Westbrook and Oliver (1991). Precisely, consumption emotions have been theorized as distinct categories of emotional experience and expressions, such as joy, anger, fear; or as a limited number of dimensions, which underlie emotional categories; and these include pleasantness/unpleasantness, relaxation/action, or calmness/excitement (Izard, 1977; Plutchik, 1980). In addition, positive emotions could lead to positive word-of-mouth behaviors, while negative emotions may cause complaining behaviors (Liljander & Strandvik, 1997). From the above, the emotional state of the consumer clearly influences how the consumer will be able to evaluate the service rendered.

### The Body Language of Both the Contact-Employee and the Customer

The behaviors exhibited by frontline service employees are vital to customer's evaluations of a service encounter (Hartline et al., 2000). Liljander and Strandvik (1995) maintain that customers who develop positive emotional responses towards individual contact employees will possess a stronger relationship with and be more committed to the service organization. Before exchanges between the customer and the contact employee are underway, the tone of the interaction can be set by the body language of both individuals. The body language is nonverbal and part of everyday social behavior, and as such, whenever one person sees another, he or she typically sees body posture, eye gaze, facial expressions, and other nonverbal cues, as asserted by Patterson (1982). "The high frequency of nonverbal behavior is consequential in that, perceivers' emotions, attitudes and behavior effortlessly respond to others' nonverbal cues" (Lamer, Reeves, & Weisbuch, 2015, p. 131).

Weisbuch and Ambady (2009) and Fromkin and Rodman (1983) propose that about 90% of the communication process occurs nonverbally. In the consumer context, Gabbott and Hogg (2000) investigated the effect of nonverbal behavior on subjects' perception of a service event. The findings indicated that nonverbal behavior, such as a high degree of direct gaze/eye contact or smiling and nodding positively affected the consumer's evaluation of the total service experience. Kleinke (1986) asserts that gaze has the tendency to influence social impressions and implications about the personality traits of individuals and leads to effects such as likeability, attractiveness, and credibility. According to a research by Droney and Brooks (1993), the longer the participants of the study looked at others in the eye, the more that participant was believed to possess positive personal qualities. This helps confirm the premise that nonverbal communication seems to be highly relevant to how consumers perceive and evaluate service (Darian, Tucci & Wiman, 2001; Kim & Kim, 2012).

## Cues and Signals of Service Quality

First, for many classes of purchases, customers have more information than ever before; this helps them to evaluate and compare possibilities and make choices among them. Alternative sources of information, such as customer review websites and social media, tend to be more trusted than advertising and communications originating from the brand, as savvy consumers know the motivations of the company. Online ratings and reviews, or "likes," and so on, serve as a democratic imperfect system, and signal to probable postpurchase satisfaction (Flanagin, Metzger, Pure, Markov, & Hartsell, 2014). The signals, thereby, inform potential buyers in a mental simulation as to their own likely satisfaction.

Second, social media also offers an outlet for the customer's voice. If a purchase is not satisfactory, customers posting complaints on company feedback boards or their own pages, might not comprise direct recompense or retribution, but customers engaged in such postings can feel more empowered and less helpless. Customers can feel that they registered their complaints to a community. And of course, some smart companies monitor their brand discussions and attend to their shortcomings (Grégoire, Salle, & Tripp, 2015).

Third, an online counterpart to third-party objective ratings, such as those continued to be offered in Consumer Reports, might be blogs by experts reporting on their trials with various goods and services and their endorsements of some options over others (Hsu, Lin, & Chiang, 2013). Blogs have strengths and weaknesses that are perfectly complementary to democratic online ratings; in particular, a blog has the advantage of often being acknowledged in expertise, but the disadvantage of, nevertheless, being only a single voice on a subject.

Fourth, other phenomena have also risen in prevalence that may be assisted by online business but can likewise arise independently. For example, marketers have always recognized price as a cue to quality, and at the nexus of price setting and service guarantees, ar  e the current phenomena of retailers' price-matching guarantees (Haruvy & Leszczyc, 2015; Yuan & Krishna, 2011); such as those offered by some large electronics and durables retailers. These guarantees are a move, which is interesting and perhaps even a bit daring, given the prevalence of online information, including frequently transparent comparative price points.

Fifth, another signal to quality is the increasing presence of co-branding, whereby one good, trusted brand name endorses or partners in some visible way with another. When Dell® and Lenovo® place stickers announcing, "Intel Inside," consumers presume that those chips must be of higher quality than a generic unnamed chip. Consumers can feel they have made a smart purchase, where extra value is obtained from purchasing a laptop with two brands on it for the price of one. In services, co-branding is exhibited when a medical center touts its affiliation with a nearby hospital, or when professional service providers build strategic directions with the support of credible consultants. One specific example is The Mayo Clinic and Arizona State University (ASU) partnership that has led to, among other things, the creation of joint education programs and the development of a Mayo Medical School campus launched in Arizona in 2017. Related to the Mayo Medical School, as part of this innovative collaboration, Mayo Medical School students take courses from ASU's graduate program in the Science of Health Care Delivery as part of their curriculum (Starr et al., 2017).

There will always be customer uncertainty in prepurchase decision-making, perhaps particularly for services, and companies and brand managers will always, therefore, struggle with how to signal their distinctive quality. Some traditional mechanisms have been challenging to continue, such as money-back guarantees, for the brand managers who fear they may well be in a losing proposition, as well as for the consumers who still struggle with how to be reimbursed and whether trying to do so will be worth the effort.

Poor business transactions are also underreported to legal or governmental Better Business Bureau sorts of associations, in part, due to consumers second-guessing themselves as to whether their experience rises to the occasion, anticipating the effort it would take to engage in the reporting and the beliefs in the likelihood of change as a result of the reporting. In addition to these opportunities for customers to "voice" their experiences, another classic mechanism is that of "exit" strategies. A consumer can exit, that is, consumers leave the product category or the brand, but this option can prove difficult in cases where a need can only be satisfied within a specific market/product category; for example, consumers still need to fly, even if they do not like their options. If customers are not satisfied with their purchases, and they are not satisfied with traditional venues for reporting that dissatisfaction, it is no surprise that they seek newer outlets, such as the posting of opinions online. Future phenomena are presumably likely to follow similar paths. Customers seek information to make purchases they care about as wisely as possible, and they seek opportunities to provide feedback, especially if the purchase experience was not as good as they had hoped or expected (and occasionally in zealous support of a good brand experience). Analogously, companies seeking customers will try to offer valid, if naturally somewhat inflated, information about their quality provision. Many vehicles for providing cues to quality exist, from prices and brand names to service guarantees and website presences (e.g., endorsements, videos, explanations, etc.) but these do not seem a stretch to suggest that current classes of cues will continue to develop, as will new classes and strategies.

## The Healthcare Service Business as a System

Grönroos (1990) suggests that a service system can be divided into an interactive, an invisible, and a supporting aspect. With the invisible aspect comprising the corporate culture, the service concept, and the business mission acting as the "guiding forces" of the service system, Grönroos (2007) in his later publication, adopted a more holistic view of the service system as "a network of activities involving a host of stakeholders." Gummesson (2008); Edvardsson (1996, 1997); and Edvardsson, Gustafsson, Sandén, and Johnson (2000), all assert that the service system consists of various subsystems and resources that function together to realize the service concept. Alter (2008); Maglio and Spohrer (2008); and Stauss, Engelmann, Kremer, and Luhn (2008) emphasize that the service system consists of a variety of actors and resources that produce service collectively. Taking cognizance of this means that for a service business, there are various elements that must interact with each other in order for the desired service to be delivered. This process of continuous interaction of these elements is what makes a service business adopt the features of a system. It must also be noted that the complexity of the service element interaction is dependent on the type of service to be rendered. An article by Leib Leventhal (2008) concluded that "services were highlighted as being distinct from products, owing to their intangibility and delivery process requirements" (p. 58). It further stated that aged care services had been seen to be even more complex, as the customers include multiple stakeholders such as the immediate family that have their own interests, concerns, and expectations to be met (2008).

Additionally, the servuction quality is another factor to consider in how a service business works as a system. Servuction refers to the production and delivery of services—the word is easily recognized as analogous to production. The word emphasizes an essential fact: Services are different from products and should not be forced to borrow terminology from the manufacturing sector. Services need to be recognized on their own terms. It is a fact that the customer is involved in the servuction process and that the service provider has less control over the environment and the behavior of the actors. In the manufacturing process, the customer is not present. How would the quality of cars be affected if customers were allowed to wander around the factory freely and intervene at their own discretion? And what would the cars cost? In servuction, the customer is very much present. In participating in the servuction, the customer helps—or complicates—the process. Consequently, servuction quality is partly the result of interaction and joint efforts between the customer and the service provider; it is the result of a division of labor. Servuction quality refers to the ability to perform a service according to specifications. If there is a gap between servuction quality (how the service is actually performed) and design quality (how it should be performed and how well the design reflects the needs of the customers), then the customer's perceived quality is at stake. If the service has not been properly designed, there are no specifications to follow, and servuction quality cannot be measured.

One of the most quoted quality strategies is, "Do it right the first time!" This is a prevention strategy. Obviously, the design stage is the very first opportunity to influence service quality; the first time to prevent systematic and repeated errors from occurring. The design should be correct in two ways. Firstly, the service should fit the customer's needs and desires. Secondly, it should be put together to make it technically feasible to perform the service and also to do it at a competitive price. It is a matter of *designed-in quality* or simply stated, design quality. Recognizing the need for service design, the practicing businessman, politician, or public servant will look for techniques and aids for execution. Such techniques are still scarce, but they are emerging. The first, suggested by Lynn Shostack is called service blueprinting (Shostack, 1981).

Service blueprinting is a systematic way of describing a service. It is a flow-chart type of blueprint that considers the interdependence among activities, people, products, and other essential parts of the servuction. The purpose of blueprinting is to make sure that all elements are there, to find out their cost and contribution to revenue, and to facilitate strategic decisions on the composition of the service. Two interesting concepts of service blueprinting are the line of visibility (what should be seen by the customer and what should not be seen) and fail points (the parts of the service which are most sensitive to errors). As an example of an application, Figure 8.4 shows a portion of a service blueprint made for Richmond Metropolitan Blood Services, a not-for-profit blood center which collects blood from volunteers and supplies it to hospitals (George & Gibson, 1991).

In conclusion, a service design strategy, especially when using a systematic approach, should do the following;

1. Give a complete overview of the service.
2. Develop strategic decisions regarding the composition of the service.
3. Analyze the cost, capital, and revenue effects of the inclusion or exclusion of service elements.
4. Analyze the weaknesses—fail points—of the servuction process to create a less accident-prone service, that is, to enhance robustness.
5. Communicate to employees, and sometimes also to customers, the total service concept and how everyone's role in the servuction process influences the outcome.
6. Incorporate inspiration from the systematic design approaches used in manufacturing industries. However, it should not force manufacturing conditions and design lessons from steel mills and pharmaceutical companies on consultancy, hairdressing or hospitals; services must be allowed to thrive on their own design conditions.
7. Remember that service design must allow for the fact that two groups are interacting in the servuction: The employees of the service provider and the customers. Sometimes a highly standardized interaction, including the use of machinery, is preferable; sometimes, each situation is highly unique and dependent on human contact.

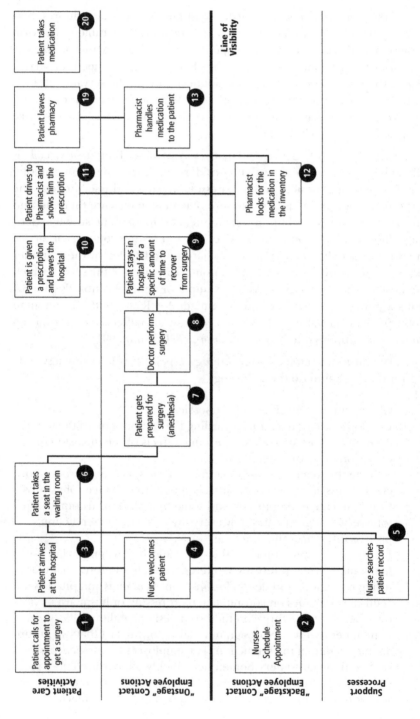

**Figure 8.4**   Service blueprint of a hospital customer service. *Source:* Kumar & Steinebach, 2008.

8. Acknowledge that individual customers—as well as employees—are different in skills, needs, mood, time pressure, honesty, and so on. The service design should allow for differences, promoting their positive effects, and minimizing their negative effects.
9. Give room in the design for the employees to act on the spur of the moment, mobilizing their personalities to solve problems in the best interest of the customer and the employer. They should be guided by both results—creating customer loyalty—and by necessary rituals and routines.

## Conclusion

Those who use healthcare facilities, privately or publicly owned, are stakeholders who are also customers of the healthcare organizations. They have a pattern of searching for information and using and evaluating healthcare providers. These are their inherent behaviors. Managers need to understand these customer behaviors to develop their marketing strategy. The chapter highlighted customer interaction with health services operation and the way this can shape the business relationship.

Customer expectations to receive quality healthcare services is also recognized in this chapter. Usually, each customer has different needs, but overall, they want good services. Efforts should be made to meet and exceed these expectations. Managers need to evaluate further how the services are being provided and need to deal with any issues or complaints as soon as they arrive. This can go a long way in creating a positive attitude and enhancing the reputation of the organization.

## Review Questions

1. Explain the health service business as a system.
2. How can customer needs and expectations be continuously monitored?
3. What are the cues and signals of quality service healthcare?

## MINI CASE STUDY: CUSTOMER EXPECTATIONS

Emmanuel Osei visited Freedom Care Clinic, Ghana, at about 1:00 a.m. with his brother, who was experiencing severe nausea and diarrhea. This clinic had been highly rated for good customer service and quality healthcare delivery, so Emmanuel had already formed a high level of expectation of his brother's treatment there.

On arrival, Emmanuel immediately observed that the waiting room and parking area were already over-taxed, and the clinic was enclosed by a restaurant on one side and a neighborhood grocery store on the other. One of the nurses looked up from her cluttered desk and snapped, "Aha, so what's wrong with him?" Astonished at her uncaring attitude, Emmanuel could only think to respond, "He's very sick and needs help." He helped his brother lay on a nearby narrow wooden bench, helpless to get the attention of unconcerned nurses until, after several minutes, a doctor came to take him to a treatment room. After several hours of treatment, his brother was released. Emmanuel was waved into the business office to settle the bills. A clerk handed him the bill and, without any form of greetings, said, "You owe us GH280. Will you pay with cash or check?"

Emmanuel had expected to have an opportunity to talk to the doctor about his brother's condition and receive some advice on what to expect. However, no such meeting was offered, even after Emmanuel asked to speak to the doctor. "He's too busy to talk to you," was all the clerk had to say. All expectations he had about Freedom Care Clinic were crushed.

### Discussion Questions

1. Using these three service quality dimensions—corporate quality (image), physical quality, and interactive quality—provide an assessment of Freedom Care Clinic in this case.
2. Assume that the doctor who had attended to Emmanuel's brother had met with him and offered some advice for further treatment, do you think Emmanuel would have left with a positive perception about the clinic regardless of the poor service he initially encountered with the nurse or clerk? Will he return to Freedom Care in the future or look for another clinic? What steps should Freedom Care take to improve their public image?

## References

Aigbavboa, C. (2016). Assessing beneficiary's needs and expectations as a determinant of residential satisfaction in South Africa. *Housing, Care and Support, 19*(1), 10–22.

Al-Kwifi, O. S., & Ahmed, Z. U. (2015). An intellectual journey into the historical evolution of marketing research in brand switching behavior—past, present and future. *Journal of Management History, 21*(2), 172–193.

Alalaakkola, L. (1996). Aged consumers as a research subject. In P. Tuominen (Ed.), *Emerging perspectives in marketing* (Series A-10). Publications of the Turku School of Economics and Business Administration, Turku.

Alter, S. (2008). Service system fundamentals: Work system, value chain and life cycle. *IBM Systems Journal, 7*(1), 71–85.

Andaleeb, S. S. (2001). Service quality perceptions and patients' satisfaction: A study of hospitals in a developing country. *Social Science & Medicine, 52*(9), 1359–1370.

Andersson, P., Wästlund, E., & Kristensson, P. (2016). The effect of gaze on consumers' encounter evaluation. *International Journal of Retail & Distribution Management, 44*(4), 372–396.

Bardwell, R. (1984), The development and motivational function of expectations. *American Education Research Journal, 21*(2), 461–472.

Berman, B. (2005). How to delight your customers. *California Management Review, 48*(1), 129–151.

Bettencourt, L. A., & Gwinner, K. (1996). Customization of the service experience: The role of the frontline employee. *International Journal of Service Industry Management, 7*(2), 3–20.

Bitner, M. J. (1990). Evaluating service encounters: The effects of physical surroundings and employee responses. *Journal of Marketing, 54*(2), 69–82.

Bitner, M. J. (1992). Servicescapes: The impact of physical surroundings on customers and employees. *Journal of Marketing, 56*(2), 57–71.

Boulding, W., Kalna, A., Staelin, R., & Zeithaml, V. A. (1993). A dynamic process model of service quality: From expectations to behavioral intentions. *Journal of Marketing Research, 30*(1), 7–27.

Bowden, J. L H. (2009). The process of customer engagement: A conceptual framework. *Journal of Marketing Theory and Practice, 17*(1), 63–74.

Chiu, H. C., & Lin, N. P. (2004). A service quality measurement derived from the theory of needs. *The Service Industries Journal, 24*(1), 187–204.

Churchill, G. A., Collins, R. H., & Strang, W. A. (1975). Should retail people be similar to their customers? *Journal of Retailing, 51,* 21–42.

Coye, R. W. (2004). Managing customer expectations in the service encounter. *International Journal of Service Industry Management, 15*(1), 54–71.

Cronin, J. J., Jr., Brady, M. K., & Hult, G. T. M. (2000). Assessing the effects of quality, value, and customer satisfaction on consumer behavioral intentions in service environments. *Journal of Retailing, 76*(2), 193–218.

Crosby, L. A., Evans, K. R., & Cowles, D. (1990). Relationship quality in services selling, an interpersonal influence perspective. *Journal of Marketing, 54*(3), 68–81.

Droney, J. M., & Brooks, C. L. (1993). Attributions of self-esteem as a function of duration of eye contact. *Journal of Social Psychology, 133*(5), 715–722.

Edvardsson, B. (1996), *Kvalitet och tjaensteutveckling*, Lund: Studentlitteratur.

Edvardsson, B. (1997). Quality in new service development: Key concepts and a frame reference. *International Journal of Production Economics, 52*(1–2), 31–46.

Edvardsson, B., Gustafsson, A., Sandén, B., & Johnson, M. D. (2000). *New service development and innovation in the new economy.* Lund, Sweden: Studenltitteratur.

Eiglier, P., & Langeard, E. (1977). *A new approach to service marketing. Marketing consumer services: New insights.* Cambridge, MA: Marketing Science Institute.

Erevelles, S., & Leavitt, C. (1992). A comparison of current models of consumer satisfaction/dissatisfaction. *Journal of Consumer Satisfaction, Dissatisfaction and Complaining Behavior, 5*(10), 104–114.

Fisk, R. P. (1981). *Toward a consumption/evaluation process model for services.* In J. H. Donnelly & W. R. George (Eds.), *Marketing of services* (pp 191–195). Chicago, IL: American Marketing Association.

Flanagin, A. J., Metzger, M. J., Pure, R., Markov, A., & Hartsell, E. (2014). Mitigating risk in ecommerce transactions: Perceptions of information credibility and the role of user-generated ratings in product quality and purchase intention. *Electronic Commerce Research, 14*(1), 1–23.

Fromkin, V., & Rodman, J. (1983). *An introduction to language.* New York, NY: CBS College.

Gabbott, M., & Hogg, G. (2000). An empirical investigation of the impact of non-verbal communication on service evaluation. *European Journal of Marketing, 34*(3/4), 384–398.

Gadel, M. S. (1964). Concentration by salesmen on congenial prospects. *Journal of Marketing, 28*(2), 64–66.

George W. R., & Gibson B. E. (1991). Blueprinting: A tool for managing quality in service's. In W. Brown et al. (Eds.), *Quality in services: Multidisciplinary and multinational perspectives* (pp. 73–91). Lexington, MA: Lexington Books.

Gilbert, F. W., Lumpkin, J. R., & Dant, R. P. (1992). Adaptation and customer expectations of health care options. *Journal of Health Care Management, 12*(3), 46–55.

Grégoire, Y., Salle, A., & Tripp, T. M. (2015). Managing social media crises with your customers: The good, the bad, and the ugly. *Business Horizons, 58*(2), 173–182.

Grönroos, C. (1982). An applied service marketing theory. *European Journal of Marketing, 16*(7), 30–41.

Grönroos, C. (1990). *Service management and marketing: Managing the moments of truth in service competition.* Lexington, MA: Lexington books.

Grönroos, C. (2001). The perceived service quality concept–a mistake? Managing service quality. *An International Journal, 11*(3), 150–152.

Grönroos, C. (2007). *Service management and marketing: Customer management in service competition* (Vol. 3). Chichester, England: Wiley.

Gummesson, E. (2008). Extending the service-dominant logic: From customer centricity to balanced centricity. *Journal of the Academy of Marketing Science, 36,* 15–17.

Gwinner, K. P., Bitner, M. J., Brown, S. W., & Kumar, A. (2005). Service customization through employee adaptiveness. *Journal of Service Research, 8*(2), 131–148.

Hartline, M., Maxham, J., & McKee, D. (2000). Corridors of influence in the dissemination of customer-oriented strategy to customer contact service employees. *Journal of Marketing, 64*(2), 35–50.

Haruvy, E., & Leszczyc, P. T. L. (2015). Measuring the impact of price guarantees on bidding in consumer online auctions. *Journal of Retailing, 92*(1), 96–108.

Helson, H. (1964). *Adaptation level theory.* New York, NY: Harper & Row.

Hsu, C. L., Lin, J. C. C., & Chiang, H. S. (2013). The effects of blogger recommendations on customers' online shopping intentions. *Internet Research, 23*(1), 69–88.

Izard, C. E. (1977). *Human emotions.* New York, NY: Plenum Press.

Kang, J., & Hillery, J. (1998). Older salespeople's role in retail encounters. *Journal of Personal Selling & Sales Management, 18*(4), 39–53.

Kano, N., Seraku, N., Takahashi, F., & Tsuji, S. (1984). Attractive quality and must-be quality. *Journal of Japanese Society for Quality Control, 14*(2), 39–48.

Kim, J. E., & Kim, J. (2012). Human factors in retail environments: A review. *International Journal of Retail & Distribution Management, 40*(11), 818–841.

Kim, M. G., & Mattila, A. S. (2013). Does a surprise strategy need words? The effect of explanations for a surprise strategy on customer delight and expectations. *Journal of Services Marketing, 27*(5), 361–370.

Kleinke, C. L. (1986). Gaze and eye contact, a research review. *Psychological Bulletin, 100*(1), 78–100.

Kumar, S., & Steinebach, M. (2008). Eliminating US hospitals medical errors. *International Journal of Health Care Quality Assurance, 21*(5), 444–471.

Lamer, S. A., Reeves, S. L., & Weisbuch, M. (2015). The nonverbal environment of self-esteem: Interactive effects of facial-expression and eye-gaze on perceivers' self-evaluation. *Journal of Experimental Social Psychology, 56,* 130–138.

Landy, F., & Trumbo, D. (1980). *Psychology of work behavior.* Homewood, IL: The Dorsey Press.

Langeard, E., Bateson, J. E., Lovelock, C. H., & Eiglier, P. (1981). *Services marketing: New insights from consumers and managers.* Cambridge, MA: Marketing Science Institute.

Leventhal, L. (2008). The role of understanding customer expectations in aged care. *International Journal of Health Care Quality Assurance, 21*(1), 50–59.

Liljander, V., & Strandvik, T. (1995). The nature of customer relationships in services. In T. A. Swartz, D. E. Bowen, & S. W. Brown (Eds.), *Advances in services marketing and management.* London, England: JAI Press.

Liljander, V., & Strandvik, T. (1997). Emotions in service satisfaction. *International Journal of Service Industry Management, 8*(2), 148–169.

Lim, P. C., Tang, N. K. H., & Jackson, P. M. (1999). An innovative framework for health care performance measurement. *Managing Services Quality, 9*(6), 423–434.

Lovelock, C., & Wirtz, J. (2011). *Services marketing: People, technology, strategy* (7th ed). Upper Saddle River, NJ: Prentice Hall.

Lusch, R. F., & Vargo, S. L. (2006, September). Service-dominant logic: Reactions, reflections, and refinements. *Marketing Theory, 6,* 281–288.

Maglio, P. P., & Spohrer, J. (2008). Fundamentals of service science. *Journal of the Academy of Marketing Science, 36,* 18–20.

Maslow, A. H. (1970). *Motivation and personality.* New York, NY: Harper and Row.

McEwen, W. (2004). Why satisfaction isn't satisfying. *Gallup Management Journal, 11.* Retrieved from https://news.gallup.com/businessjournal/14023/Why-Satisfaction-Isnt-Satisfying.aspx

Mills, P. K., Chase, R. B., & Marguiles, N. (1983). Motivating the client/employee system as a service production strategy. *Academy of Management Review, 8*(2), 301–310.

Newcomb, T. M. (1956). The prediction of interpersonal attraction. *American Psychologist, 11*(11), 575–586.

Noone, B. M., & Mattila, A. S. (2009). Consumer reaction to crowding for extended service encounters. *Managing Service Quality, 19*(1), 31–41.

Oliver, R. L. (1980). Theoretical bases of consumer satisfaction research: Review, critique and future direction. In W. L. Charles & M. D. Patrick (Eds.), *Theoretical developments in marketing* (pp. 206–210). Chicago, IL: American Marketing Association.

Oliver, R. L. (1997). *Satisfaction: A behavioral perspective on the consumer.* New York, NY: McGrawHill.

Oliver, R. L., Rust, R. T., & Varki, S. (1997). Customer delight: Foundations, findings, and managerial insight. *Journal of Retailing, 73*(3), 311–336.

Parasuraman, A., Zeithaml, V. A., & Berry, L. L. (1985). A conceptual model of service quality and its implications for future research. *Journal of Marketing, 49*(4), 41–50.

Parasuraman, A., Zeithaml, V. A., & Berry, L. L. (1988). SERVQUAL: A multiple-item scale for measuring customer perceptions of service quality. *Journal of Retailing, 64*(1), 12–37.

Patterson, M. L. (1982). A sequential functional model of nonverbal exchange. *Psychological Review, 89*(3), 231–249.

Plutchik, R. (1980). *Emotion: A psychoevolutionary synthesis.* New York, NY: Harper and Row.

Reisig, D. M., & Chandek, M. S. (2001). The effects of expectancy disconfirmation on outcome satisfaction in police-citizen encounters. *An International Journal of Police Strategies & Management, 24*(1), 88–99.

Santos, J., & Boote, J. (2003). A theoretical exploration and model of consumer expectations, post-purchase affective states and affective behavior. *Journal of Consumer Behavior, 3*(2), 142–156.

Schiffman, L. G., & Kanuk, L. L. (2007). *Purchasing behavior.* Upper Saddle River, NJ: Pearson Prentice Hall.

Schneider, B., & Bowen, D. E. (1995). *Winning the service game.* Boston, MA: Harvard Business School Press.

Shostack, L. G. (1985). Planning the service encounter. In J. A. Czepiel, M. R. Solomon, & C. F. Surprenant (Eds.), *The service encounter* (pp. 243–254). Lexington, MA: Lexington Books.

Solomon, M., Surprenant, C., Czepiel, J., & Gutman, E. (1985). A role theory perspective on dyadic interactions: The service encounter. *Journal of Marketing, 49*(1), 99–111.

Spreng, R., MacKenzie, S., & Olshavsky, R. (1996). A re-examination of the determinants of consumer satisfaction. *Journal of Marketing, 60*(3), 15–32.

Starr, S. R., Agrwal, N., Bryan, M. J., Buhrman, Y., Gilbert, J., Huber, J. M., . . . Patel, A. M. (2017). Science of health care delivery: An innovation in undergraduate medical education to meet society's needs. *Mayo Clinic Proceedings: Innovations, Quality & Outcomes, 1*(2), 117–129.

Stauss, B., Engelmann, K., Kremer, A., & Luhn, A. (Eds). (2008). *Service science: Fundamentals, challenges and future developments.* Berlin, Germany: Springer.

Stauss, B., & Neuhaus, P. (1997). The qualitative satisfaction model. *International Journal of Service Industry Management, 8*(3), 236–249.

Sujan, H., Weitz, B. A., & Kumar, N. (1994). Learning orientation, working smart, and effective selling. *Journal of Marketing, 58*(3), 39–52.

Tse, D. K., & Wilton, P. C. (1988). Models of consumer satisfaction formation: An extension. *Journal of Marketing Research, 25*(2), 204–212.

Tsiotsou, R. H., & Wirtz, J. (2012). Consumer behavior in a service context. In V. Wells & G. Foxall (Eds.), *Handbook of developments in consumer behavior* (pp. 147–201). Cheltenham, MA: Edward Elgar.

Vogenberg, F., Santilli, J. (2018). Healthcare trends for 2018. *American Health Drug Benefits, 11*(1), 48–54.

Wägar, K., & Lindqvist, L. J. (2010). The role of the customer contact person's age in service encounters. *Journal of Services Marketing, 24*(7), 509–517.

Walker, J. L. (1995). Service encounter satisfaction conceptualized. *Journal of Services Marketing, 9*(1), 5–14.

Weisbuch, M., & Ambady, N. (2009). Unspoken cultural influence: Exposure to and influence of nonverbal bias. *Journal of Personality and Social Psychology, 96*(6), 1104–1119.

Weitz, B. A., Sujan, H., & Sujan, M. (1986). Knowledge, motivation, and adaptive behavior: A framework for improving selling effectiveness. *Journal of Marketing, 50*(4), 174–191.

Westbrook, R. A., & Oliver, R. L. (1991). The dimensionality of consumption emotion patterns and consumer satisfaction. *Journal of Consumer Research, 18*(1), 84–91.

Wirth, J. H., Sacco, D. F., Hugenberg, K., & Williams, K. D. (2010). Eye gaze as relational evaluation: Averted eye gaze leads to feelings of ostracism and relational devaluation. *Personality and Social Psychology Bulletin, 36*(7), 869–882.

Wong, A. (2004). The role of emotional satisfaction in service encounters. *Managing Service Quality: An International Journal, 14*(5), 365–376.

Woodruff, R., Cadotte, E., & Jenkins, R. (1983). Modeling consumer satisfaction processes using experience-based norms. *Journal of Marketing Research, 20*(3), 296–304.

Yuan, H., & Krishna, A. (2011). Price-matching guarantees with endogenous search: a market experiment approach. *Journal of Retailing, 87*(2), 182–193.

Zeithaml, V. A., Berry, L. L., & Parasuraman, A. (1993). The nature and determinants of customer expectations of service. *Journal of the Academy of Marketing Science, 21*(1), 1–12.

# 9

## *Positioning Healthcare Services in Competitive Markets*

### Chapter Outline

- Introduction
- Focus Strategy and Competitive Advantage
- Service Differentiation Variables
- Internal, Market, and Competitor Analysis
- Dimensions of Marketing Analysis
- Positioning Maps
- How to Effect Changes in Competitive Positioning
- Competitive Analysis
- Conclusion
- Review Questions
- Mini Case Study With Discussion Questions
- References

*Marketing in Healthcare-Related Industries,* pages 205–225
Copyright © 2020 by Information Age Publishing
All rights of reproduction in any form reserved.

## Chapter Outcome

By the end of this chapter, the reader will be able to

- explain how focus underlies the search for competitive advantage;
- understand market segmentation as the basis for focused strategies;
- explain how positioning distinguishes a brand from its competitors;
- discuss internal, market, and competitor analyses in relation to service delivery;
- explain how service institutions use positioning maps to plot competitive strategy; and
- describe how competitive positioning can be changed.

## Introduction

To succeed in competitive markets and overcommunicated societies, a health service company must create a position in the prospect's mind that takes into consideration not only its own strengths and weaknesses, but also those of its competitors. A company must be focused on creating, communicating, and maintaining some uniqueness, which will be detected and valued by those with whom it intends to develop a long-term relationship. This requires managers to understand their target customer's preferences and their competitors. Having a strategic focus is a common characteristic of successful organizations. However, different schools of thought exist about how companies can use strategy to gain a competitive advantage over competitors.

## Focus Strategy and Competitive Advantage

According to Porter's (1980) argument on competition, firms can pursue generic strategies to achieve a better competitive position in the marketplace by combining two elements: the field (a company's decision to extend activities) and the type of competitive advantage (a firm's decision method on how to develop a competitive advantage). However, the strategy selection process cannot be generically condensed and unified. This is because each company's profitability is dependent on the ability to design and implement the strategy which has the potential of leading to the growth of the company. Firms who are market leaders in an industry do not consider that operating in a niche market could be beneficial to their success. It can be costly or difficult for multi-segment competitors to put capabilities in place to meet the specialized needs of buyers. The focus strategy was also developed by Porter (1985) and is employed when a company aims to serve the customers in a narrow market segment by adopting low cost or differentiation strategies (Porter, 1980). Thompson, Strickland, Gamble, and Zeng'an Gao (2008), as a build-up of Porter's competitive strategies, indicate that the focus strategy is attractive in niche markets only when such a market is big enough to make a profit and at the same time, allow the firm to satisfy the expectations of mainstream customers. Different niches or market segments exist in the service sector. This provides the opportunity for service firms pursuing the focus strategy to select a niche that is competitively attractive so that their resources, strengths, and capabilities can be used to satisfy customers. Adopting the differentiation or low-cost competitive strategies offer firms the chance to generate higher profits.

The emphasis of the focus strategy is that of operating in a narrow market in which the firm makes efforts to be the cost leader or can achieve differentiation. The focus strategy is based on the premise that an organization can better serve the needs and wants of a group of people or a market segment if it concentrates on these entirely. One benefit organizations gain from adopting the focus strategy is high levels of customer loyalty. Consequently, other firms in the industry often dread competing directly with firms that adopt the focus strategy. Again, firms pursuing the focus strategy, accurately differentiate and capitalize on the nonavailability of substitute goods or services to pass higher costs onto customers. However, due to the narrow nature of their markets, firms that pursue the focus strategy have lower volumes of production and, hence, have less bargaining power when dealing with suppliers. The success of the focus strategy is based on the organizations' ability to make tailor-made products that suit the needs of consumers in a narrow market, and this can be achieved by knowing the customer. However, imitation and change of markets remain some risks of a focus strategy. Further, it might not be a difficult task for a cost leader in a broader market to alter its products to compete with firms in narrow markets. Nonetheless, other "focusers" may be able to carve out subsegments so that they can serve even better.

To achieve high levels of performance, successful companies leverage competitive advantages in the marketplace, either by differentiating themselves from competitors or from lead market segments where their efforts are focused (Markgraf, n.d.). Focus strategy clearly identifies particular market segments where the company can effectively and successfully compete (Markgraf, n.d.). The strategy is in line with market characteristics, with the company's competitive advantages to identify, plan, and strategize on markets where the focus of the company's resources will likely result in desired sales volumes, revenues, and profits (Markgraf, n.d.).

### Cost

Low cost of production could be a great strategy to leverage competitive advantage, but it may not always be applicable to all markets (Markgraf, n.d.), including healthcare. The key is to segment a company market into sections that can reach customers that are cost-sensitive. Once the company has identified market segments in which consumers are looking for the lowest prices, then the company can use a focus strategy to concentrate its resources there. Ideally, the cost of reaching those consumers is low, allowing the company to maintain its price advantage while focusing on increasing sales. This focus strategy is applicable in industries such as the hospitality industry where pricing is critical to branding. However, price is not a major element in competition in healthcare, it is always difficult to capitalize cost advantage because there is a lack of price transparency. For instance, health insurance companies have become oligopolistic markets; they generally do not engage in price competition in the United States.

### Quality

Some consumers prefer to pay more to get better quality of service. If the company has a superior design, more expertise, or provides better quality of goods or services, the company may have a competitive advantage on service quality. In this case, the company has to identify market segments that will buy its higher-priced products or services. Focus strategy lets the company concentrate promotional resources on the sectors that match the company's quality advantage. Since the company is no longer competing at a low price, it can cover the higher costs involved in identifying and reaching these high-value segments. Service quality is gradually becoming the most important tool for healthcare providers to create competitive advantages. Hospital marketers should strive to create and maintain a positive brand image in order to enhance service quality, patient satisfaction, and loyalty (Wu, 2011). For healthcare providers, the best approach in differentiating their services would be to deliver consistently higher quality services than their competitors (Kemp, Jillapalli, & Becerra, 2014).

### Brand

If the company's competitive advantage includes selling a well-known brand, the company has to use focus strategy to make sure the firm is reaching the consumers who have a positive image of the brand, who need the service, and who can afford to buy it. Although some brands traverse many market segments, others such as sports-related brands, require more focus (Markgraf, n.d.). Focus strategy for brands involves targeting promotional activities to create awareness for the target consumers that are likely to be interested in the brand (Markgraf, n.d.). One way of achieving this is by engaging in corporate social responsibility activities, as this can help establish effective commitment in consumer-brand relationships in a healthcare context (Kemp et al., 2014). Brand image, service quality, trust, customer satisfaction, relationship commitment, brand loyalty, and brand awareness are major factors affecting healthcare branding (Chahal & Bala, 2012; Kim, Kim, Kim, Kim, & Kang, 2008).

## *Service*

Companies that compete on service can achieve competitive advantage by focusing on customer satisfaction. In this case, the companies channel more resources on customer service and attainment of customer satisfaction (Markgraf, n.d.). These efforts entail hiring highly skilled employees with good people skills, training them in customer relations, in the brand's products and also to monitor how swift their response time is (Markgraf, 2019). These efforts entail hiring highly skilled employees with good people skills, training them in customer relations and in the brand's products, and monitoring how swift their response time is (Markgraf, 2019).

While variation in profitability across industries explains why some firms are more profitable than others, the variation in profitability among players within the same industry is even more striking. For Porter (1985), the explanation is to be found in the relative effectiveness of their strategy. The primary aim of strategy is to be different rather than better. For instance, better operational effectiveness can indeed confer a temporary advantage, but this is much more easily matched by competitors than is a distinctive strategic positioning. To replicate a strategy, competitors will have to change their methods in ways that are likely to leave them in conflict.

## *Technology*

Technology can affect competitive advantage if it has a significant role in determining relative cost or differentiation (Porter, 1985). Increasingly, as technology is utilized in most business activities, both in the production and dissemination of products and services, it can also have a great effect on both cost and differentiation. However, through technology, a firm can successfully gain a more competitive advantage if able to discover, create, or utilize a technology that surpasses that of its competitors in performing its activities. Apart from affecting cost or differentiation, technology also affects the competitive advantage through changing or influencing the other drivers of cost or uniqueness. Technology has profoundly changed the healthcare landscape. Healthcare organizations are increasingly adopting and promoting cutting-edge and sophisticated technologies to differentiate themselves from competitors and to build a sustainable competitive advantage. The use of technology increases the provider's capabilities and the patients' access to healthcare and improves the structure and processes of healthcare delivery, which ultimately enhances the quality of care and the quality of life for some patients (Skinner, 2017). Research suggests that hospitals that invest more extensively in clinical technologies tend to be better performers, regardless of location (Goldstein, Ward, Leong, & Butler, 2002). Technology can help healthcare organizations reduce costs, but increased use of new medical technology also contributes to rising healthcare costs.

### Market Segmentation

The concept of market segmentation is often cited as crucial to establishing a target market strategy (Kotler & Keller, 2005; Simkin, 2008). Market segmentation involves grouping customers so that those in one segment share common characteristics, purchasing behavior, needs, usage and attitudes, which are reasonably homogenous, while other customers who share a different set of traits and behaviors are allocated to a separate market segment (Bonoma & Shapiro, 1984; Engel, Fiorillo, & Cayley, 1972; Weinstein, 2004; Simkin, 2008). There are various approaches to creating market segments including survey-based quantitative studies of customer behavior or more ad-hoc qualitative approaches such as intuitively interpreting sentiments expressed during customer focus groups, to the macro–micro evolution, to newly defined segments based on assessing existing customer groupings or classifications. In creating market segments, this approach also develops a better understanding of customers, which is a rather crucial requisite for effective marketing (Vandermerwe, 2004). This process also engenders commitment from the managers responsible for implementing the eventual segmentation scheme.

Segmentation enables an organization selectively to target "good" business (Anderson & Narus, 2003; Dibb, Stern, & Wensley, 2002). Weinstein (2004) argues a persuasive case for practicing market segmentation, which is not the purpose of this discourse. Here, the focus is on outlining a means of developing segments while minimizing internal resistance to the associated change.

Since the goal of a marketing strategy is to identify a target market and develop a marketing mix to appeal to potential customers, it is important to consider the right marketing mix that will appeal to your identified target audience (Hopps, n.d.). The adoption of the technique of market segmentation; of understanding the characteristics of customer/user needs, using one or more bases either singly or in combination; and that of market targeting, selecting one or more of the identified segments as the basis for the development of a competitive strategy, are indisputable for any organization faced with the application of limited resources in attempting to achieve its objectives. This applies whether the objectives are strategic (an acceptable return on the capital employed) and/or tactical (increase in market share or sales revenue).

Market segmentation is a concept which seeks to group existing and potential customers into segments which have similar attitudes and characteristics and are likely to subscribe to the same product. Thus, segments contain relatively homogeneous customers but are different from other (heterogeneous) segments. The advantages, as stated by Engel, Fiorillo, and Cayley (1972) are

- the efficient allocation of resources,
- the ability to recognize and capitalize on opportunities, and
- greater customer satisfaction and loyalty.

For both personal and business customers, there is, however, a plethora of bases which may be considered when trying to segment the total market. These range from the quantitative (i.e., demographic, economic, size, and type of customer) to the qualitative (i.e., psychographic, behavioral, benefit sought) and may be used singly or in some form of combination. Healthcare organizations usually use demographic (e.g., age, income, gender, ethnicity, family size) and geographic (e.g., region, location) segmentation approaches. They can also benefit from using psychological (e.g., lifestyles, personality traits, beliefs, values, attitudes, interests) and behavioral (e.g., purchase, use) segmentation strategies.

## Positioning

In an era of hyper-competition, competitive differentiation is at the heart of marketing strategy. In light of this, several healthcare organizations are leveraging on brand extensions as a strategy for competitive differentiation. Unfortunately, these brand extensions often fail to achieve the intended purpose due to lack of uniqueness and its subsequent inability to appeal to consumers. Consequently, engaging in brand extensions poses financial risks. In recent times, the financial burden in creating brand extensions has increased due to increased cost in distribution and promotional activities (Smith & Park, 1992). For a brand extension to succeed as a differentiation strategy, it must embed unique characteristics that offer exceptional value to consumers. Regardless of the failure of most brand extensions to serve as differentiated products, the concept still provides a means through which firms can gain brand equity. One advantage of leveraging on a strong parent brand to introduce new products is the reduction in the risk involved in introducing an entirely new brand on an existing market. A major drawback to competitive differentiation via brand extensions is that the extended brands often promise to be new, bigger, and better than the existing ones and which they fail to do. However, more often, competitive differentiation emerges from the organization creating value that is above the consumer's expectations (Albert, Merunka, & Valette-Florence, 2008). In efforts to differentiate products, most brand extensions end up being similar to each other or with the parent brand, thereby, failing to achieve the objectives (McGovern & Moon, 2007). Organizations, therefore, can achieve commoditization of the extended brands by adding new features to them. In these instances, the main focus of competitive differentiation is brand positioning. To ensure a unified positioning strategy, critical strategic decisions must be taken by brand managers with regards to brand extension.

Brand positioning refers to the perception of consumers about a brand relative to specific vital brand attributes, benefits, and values (Keller, 2008). It is the summation of the perceptions, impressions, and feelings consumers hold towards a brand (Brooksbank, 1994). The perception the consumer embraces about a brand is based on the unique view he or she has in mind about the brand, relative to competing brands. Therefore, brand positioning is based on two factors: how consumers perceive the brand, and the brand's position relative to competitors. In the end, the consumer is the decider of the effectiveness of brand positioning. Hence, the focus of a brand positioning strategy should be differentiation. Typically, a differentiation strategy is grounded on the product itself, the brand image, on employees, on services provided, and distribution channels used (Kotler & Keller, 2006). Every differentiation strategy should be fixated on realizing the means-end chain of attributes, benefits, and values. Differentiation strategies that relate to goods mostly rely on intrinsic attributes of the products such as style, design, durability, reliability, reparability, functional characteristics, or structural performance. For instance, whereas Unilever places much emphasis on the functional characteristics of its products, its competitor, P&G, focuses on reliability and structural performance.

Service firms can achieve differentiation through the provision of better overall services like installation, consulting, repairs, and customer training. For instance, Southwest Airlines, in its quest to achieve differentiation, provides exclusive services to consumers through customization. Beyond achieving product differentiation, a company can also rely on service differentiation to distinguish themselves from the competition. By offering more value-adding services as well as by improving its quality, a company can differentiate its offer based on services. There are situations when companies have little scope for differentiating the tangible product. In such situations, a company can pursue the policy of service differentiation. Some of the important service differentiation variables are ease of ordering, delivery, installation, training of customers on product usage, customer consulting, maintenance, and repair.

## Service Differentiation Variables

**Ordering Ease:** It relates to the convenience or comfort that customers enjoy while ordering the product. There are companies that offer customers facilities to order products sitting at home with the punch of a computer button. There are other companies that either send their salespeople regularly to customers' doorsteps to collect orders or phone them to receive orders.

**Delivery:** The process of delivery is known as distribution, and it involves both the selection of suitable channels for distribution and the physical movement of items associated with the marketing of the product. Delivery is an important means of differentiation of a company's service. Customers prefer prompt and timely delivery, and a company can build its image as a fast and timely deliverer of products.

The brand position develops a competitive advantage that will distinguish the company's offerings from those of its competitors in the segment. In other words, the firm must decide how the business is going to compete in the marketplace. The aim is to make a unique offer to the customer, so they will be less likely to switch to competitors for minor price advantages. When developing a competitive advantage, the essential factors are delivering value to the customer beyond favorable pricing and sustainability of the differentiation strategy. In other words, it should exploit the skills of the company that competitors do not have and cannot easily imitate.

## Internal, Market, and Competitor Analysis

Market analysis can be conceptualized as a qualitative or quantitative evaluation of a market. Market analysis reviews the size of a market in terms of volume and value. It also assesses the different segments of markets, buying patterns, competition, and barriers to entry and regulations. A marketing analysis is conducted in order for businesses to be able to formulate a strategy on how to run your business. It is important to take into consideration certain factors in conducting a marketing analysis. One of the most important factors to consider is the use of the SWOT (strengths, weakness, opportunites, threats) analysis.

### *Dimensions of Marketing Analysis*

There are certain dimensions examined to perform a marketing analysis. These dimensions assist a company in understanding the market in which they operate. These dimensions include

- market size,
- growth rate of the market,
- market trends,
- market profitability,
- key success factors,
- distribution channels, and
- industry cost structure.

### *Internal Analysis*

Internal analysis is done by identifying and assessing some precise characteristics of an organization. Aside from the assessment of specific characteristics, internal assessment also covers identifying and evaluating an organization's

- resources,
- capabilities,
- core competencies,
- current vision,
- mission,
- strategic objectives, and
- strategies.

Resources relate to the assets an organization uses in carrying out the activities and processes that are key to achieving what the organization was set-up to do, as well as its goals and objectives. Commonly, the resources of an organization include

- financial resources,
- physical assets,
- human resources,
- intangible resources, and
- structure-cultural resources.

Organizational resources must be effectively processed or utilized to extract value out of them. The various resources are the inputs for organizational capabilities. Organizational capabilities represent a complex and coordinated network of organizational routines and procedures that are responsible for influencing the extent to which the organization can transform its inputs (resources) into outputs (products and services).

Strategic objectives depict the foundation that sustains business and helps it in identifying the direction it is heading towards. These objectives clearly spell out the intentions of the business as well as how to mitigate weaknesses and how to promote its current operations. In mapping out a good strategy, the business is able to cater to areas like employees, customers, and the financial health of the company, among others.

The mission is a twin of vision. While vision creates a vivid image of the direction of the business, a mission communicates it. A mission statement should provide a clear statement of the purpose, the product, the geographical location, and the primary customers of the company. In clarity, the message is rightly communicated to all and creates a better understanding and motivation.

Distinctive organizational capabilities refer to the unique capabilities that an organization relies on to distinguish itself from rival firms. Organizational capabilities enable firms to out-perform competitors by building sustainable competitive advantages. An organization's capabilities are distinctive if they do the following:

- add to superior customer value that leads to obtaining real (measurable) benefits to customers,
- become difficult for competitors to imitate or duplicate, and
- permit the organization to use its capabilities in a variety of ways.

An organization's core competency represents its major value-creating abilities and capabilities which extend across the different business sections or product lines of the firm. The shared nature of core competency within the organization is what differentiates it from distinctive capabilities. The concepts of organizational capabilities, distinctive organizational capabilities, and core competencies can be distinguished based on the following:

- Core competencies are achieved through organizational capabilities.
- All organizations have organizational processes and routines to get work done.
- The combination of an organization's several capabilities creates major value-creating skills.
- The establishment of an organization's core competencies leads to the improvement and enhancement of its capabilities as well as a contribution to the development of certain distinctive organizational capabilities.

With a good mix of resources, capabilities, core competencies, the right vision, mission, strategic objectives, and strategies, an organization can achieve sustainable competitive advantage. Additionally, the organization must possess the flexibility to create, synthesize, and modify these said abilities (resources) in periods of rapid social, technological, and environmental changes.

### Competitor Analysis

The competitor analysis provides a comprehensive overview of the competitors' strengths and weaknesses as compared to the health service firm's own capabilities. This is formulated to take into account the competitors' likely actions and responses. Hence, the strategist must be able to understand a situation from the perspective of the competitor in order to appropriately predict competitor responses as well as to determine the actual outcomes of the competitors' strategic choices. They must be able to

- estimate the outcome of potential changes in strategy by a competitor;
- predict how each competitor is likely to respond to relevant strategic moves made by other firms in the industry; and
- understand how competitors in the industry will probably react to changes in key industry and environmental regulations.

What then, is the essence of competitor analysis? In view of the intricacies and depth of competitor analysis, certain simple and basic practical questions should be considered. Typical of these are:

- Which competitors do our strategies affect?
- Which moves has our strategy always countered?

In competitive analysis, it is also important to identify potential competitors. The process starts by identifying firms for whom the various barriers to entry into the industry are low or easily surmountable.

## Positioning Maps

Positioning mapping is a diagrammatical technique used by asset marketers that attempts to visually display the perceptions of customers or potential customers. Typically, the position of a health service organization's product, brand, or product line is dependent on their competition. There are often two dimensions of market maps, also known as perceptual maps. They can, however, also be multidimensional. Market maps can be used to identify existing gaps in the market, potential partners, perceived problems with the organization's product, and targets.

Positioning denotes the perception consumers have about an organization's product, relative to that of competitors. A positioning map is a graphical device to study and analyze the positions or perception of each group of competing products in respect of two specific product characteristics. It is a graph that depicts the strengths of a product based on two product characteristics labeled on the x- and y-axis. For example, to ascertain the relative positioning of different brands of cars on consumer perception about their superiority in styling and technical features, the positioning map may depict the styling attractiveness of the model along the x-axis and its technical superiority along the y-axis. Then each of the models will be plotted on a graph depending on the evaluation of customer perception of these two characteristics.

Through positioning maps, an organization can categorize existing market products in order to target each category with different positioning categories. This knowledge can be used by organizations in diverse ways. For example, it identifies the products which are the closest competitors of the company's product and the strengths and weaknesses of the company's product in respect of its competing products. It can also help the company to identify market segments with specific product requirements where they could potentially launch their new products.

Positioning maps are used by healthcare organizations in developing a market-positioning strategy for goods or services. Positioning maps are also known as perceptual maps because they are based on the perception of the consumer. Positioning maps give an organization an understanding of the positioning of existing products to decide a better market position for its products. Using this information, firms can either fill the gaps in the market with new products or find existing products in a market and compete. Perceptual mapping helps organizations understand who their customers are, where they are, how they buy, why they buy, among others. If a company has an unfavorable positioning in the minds of customers, research can then be carried out from there to ascertain the reasons for such assessments and what could be done to dispel such unsatisfactory perceptions. Perceptual mapping also enables organizations to know what consumers think about other brands, especially competitor brands. The regular usage of perceptual mapping enhances a firm's ability to track consumer preferences and change in tastes as they occur. Definition of market segments can also be done through perceptual mapping by indicating a cluster of businesses. A business can classify its potential partners or probable businesses within the clusters established in perceptual maps that might merge, since the grouping of brands indicates similarities in business attributes. Perceptual maps aid in the identification of gaps in markets where new goods and services could be introduced as well as track how the new product is being viewed in the marketplace. It is important to note that the success of a firm's marketing efforts is linked to its alignment with the business' principal goal for positioning.

The process of mapping and analysis can, at times, be unsystematic and unstable. As such, people who are engaged in the mapping process or analysis need new tools that can be used to systematically analyze their organizations' positions in hypercompetitive markets, as well as the positions of competitors. To achieve this, there is a need to track the relationship between prices and the key benefit of a product over a period of time. It is, however, not easy to appreciate benefits or prices. According to a survey by Stativity, a global research firm, in 2004, the majority of consumers are unable to specify the features of products that define the prices they are willing to pay for those products. Surprisingly, about 50% of salespeople did not the attributes that justified the prices of the goods and services they were marketing (D'Aveni, 2007).

In the health service sector, it is challenging for organizations to identify their competitive positions, because health service consumers often do not know what they are buying, and the organizations do not fully comprehend what they are charging for. Often, when senior executives of health institutions are queried on the key competitors of their organizations, they end up being unable to identify them. Some executives of healthcare organizations often describe the offering of their firms on the price-benefit map. It appears that only a limited number of healthcare executives genuinely understand the offering of their organizations; they, however, often overrate their product offering while underrating that of competitors.

## How to Effect Changes in Competitive Positioning

In today's fast-paced economy, change is a constant denominator; when faster companies are able to respond to such changes, their chances of success are higher. Hence, the ability to respond and adapt quickly to market changes can be a great source of competitive advantage. Competitive positioning is very important in every organization, because it is the means by which products and services can be differentiated from one another and so, give consumers a reason to buy. Positioning has two fundamental aspects: (a) the brand offerings which include the physical attributes, the functionality, and capability; and (b) the manner in which a brand is communicated to the target audience and how the target audience perceives the brand relative to competing brands. In order to succeed in the environment, a health service firm's positioning can change based on intense competition. For example, patients' preference is shifting from inpatient care to ambulatory care. To address this change, it is important that hospitals focus on convenience and accessibility of care and invest in outpatient facilities for their survival and growth. Positioning denotes the place that a brand occupies in the mind of the customer, compared to competitors' products. To position products or brands, companies may utilize the marketing mix to emphasize the distinguishing features of a brand or create a desired image in the mind of the target audience. Once a health service brand has achieved a strong position, it can become difficult to reposition it. Competitive positioning can be changed on the following factors: the market profile, customer segments, and competitive analysis.

### *Market Profile*

In order to assess a company's competitive positioning, the firm needs to pay close attention to the operating market profile, which encompasses the market size, competitors, and stage of growth. This helps a company realize that the marketing environment is not static, and it must thus provide itself with a fair idea of how the company can position itself well. For example, if a small private hospital is evaluating whether to expand a cardiology department with state-of-art technology, the hospital has to create a market profile by determining the size and characteristics of target patients and forecast its future market share.

---

### Customer Segments

Customer segmentation is a relevant marketing tool. When implemented rightly, the organization will benefit enormously from it. Several segments of a market are available to select from, but there are only a few that the customers of health organizations fit into. For this reason, selecting segments and placing customers must be done with precision. The precise customer segments can then be used to improve product marketing efforts, and, ultimately, profitability. Customer segmentation is a useful tool for organizations that have several customers, and that interact with them differently. Customer segmentation allows firms to recognize different customer groups consisting of people with similar needs and wants so that they can direct their resources at satisfying them perfectly. In the context of small businesses, there may be no need to segment customers, particularly if they serve a small number of customers that are easy to manage. Customer segmentation is, however, essential to businesses with a large pool of customers. Data can be derived from customer purchases, such as purchase amounts, addresses, items purchased, and payment methods, and these may be utilized as segmentation tools and services to help group customers. Services exist that can assist in profiling a customer base that can be categorized into value and lifestyle groups. Placing customers in such groups allows a company to target them better when marketing their products or services. Companies should also use customer segmentation to categorize groups of prospective customers in order to think strategically on how to address new prospects' needs and wants.

To succeed in a competitive market, healthcare providers should use appropriate market segmentation strategies to optimize the fit between their services and the consumers who receive them (Ross, Steward, & Sinacore, 1993). Like other industries, healthcare marketers can use geographic, demographic, psychographic, benefits, and behavioral segmentation methods. Healthcare firms usually segment patients based on age, income, location, insurance status, medical conditions, and health status. Healthcare providers can benefit from applying customer segmentation techniques such as predictive modeling, exploratory factor analysis, conjoint analysis and cluster analysis. For example, Moschis and Friend (2008) employed the *gerontographic segmentation technique* (a segmentation model based on aging processes and life circumstances) to segment mature consumers with respect to healthcare products and services. They used factor and cluster analyses and identified four segments (healthy hermits, ailing outgoers, frail reclusives, and healthy indulgers).

## Competitive Analysis

Competitive analysis provides the best alternative tool for organizations to assess their strengths and weaknesses against that of competitors. Conducting a competitive analysis requires the strategist to be knowledgeable about the strengths and weaknesses of the competitor, the strategist's own capabilities, and the needs and wants of consumers. Competitive analysis involves the gathering and analysis of useful information about a competitor that will be relevant in the strategy development process. The starting point of competitor analysis is the development of the objectives that it seeks to achieve. Hereafter, important competitor information is identified, information is gathered, and analysis and interpretation of information are done. By analyzing competitors, the organization will be able to formulate competitive strategy that considers the likely competitor's actions and responses. In practical terms, the strategists need to live in the competitor's strategic shoes. Competitive analysis can help healthcare managers and marketers by providing invaluable information and insight into the current state and future opportunities and gain competitive advantage over its rivals.

## Conclusion

Sustainable competitive advantage in the service sector demands alignment of the company's vision and strategic planning to meet performance goals. In conclusion, every service organization must have a unique competitive position for the company, have activities tailored to its strategy, clear trade-offs and choices vis-à-vis competitors, and establish a fit that reaches across activities. Indeed, sustainability comes not from the existence of these many parts, but from them working together in a cohesive activity system.

## Review Questions

1. Explain how focus underlies the search for competitive advantage.
2. Describe your understanding of market segmentation as the basis for focused strategies.
3. Explain how positioning distinguishes a brand from its competitors.
4. Discuss internal market and competitor analyses in relation to service delivery.

## MINI CASE STUDY: ATTRACTING THE RIGHT CUSTOMERS/PATIENTS

Westville Hospital is situated in a semi-urban community in Nigeria populated by families and individuals living a low- to middle-income lifestyle. The popular 15-year-old hospital has provided quality services at affordable prices for people within that community. The medical director, Dr. Samuel Ogunsanya, realized the hospital could attract upscale patients given its diagnostic equipment and excellent healthcare staff. He took this idea to Jude, an experienced marketing consultant, explaining that he wanted to target patients who would benefit from the high quality of care his practice offered.

Jude described a marketing strategy known as the 4Ps: place, product, price, and promotion. Dr. Ogunsanya took Jude's advice and applied them to his goal. He started with the place. He began by taking a good look at the hospital's physical facility, looking critically for areas that needed to be improved. He saw that the paint on both the interior and exterior of the building were faded and peeling; the hospital signboard was rusty, weeds had taken over the flower beds, and the flowers themselves needed care; the furniture at the front desk and in the waiting rooms were in a state of great disrepair, and the beds in the wards were old and uncomfortable. The last work that had been done on the hospital building or its furnishings was over seven years ago. While the administration devoted attention to buying updated technology and diagnostic equipment, Dr. Ogunsanya could see that despite its record of excellence in medical practice or how good the healthcare equipment was, upscale patients would not be able to see past the shabby appearance of the building.

Dr. Ogunsanya worked with his administrative staff to prepare a budget for improvements. Soon professional artisans arrived to refurbish the environment. The furniture was replaced with modern tables, chairs, lighting, and artwork. Horticulturists tore out the sad looking gardens and planted lush bushes and greenery that would require less day-to-day attention. The outside walls were painted white, and the shutters, trim, and signs were given a shiny coat of blue paint. All these renovations and refurbishing were done within two weeks. The Westville Hospital was totally transformed. "The 'place' is now set to attract the upscale customers," Dr. Ogunsanya said.

Dr. Ogunsanya was happy with the new surroundings but realized that many people dislike going to a doctor, that it would take more than a beautiful environment to see real improvement in business operations and the bottom line. He turned to the second P, product, which in this case was exemplary medical care. He could see that by personalizing the healthcare environment, patients in a higher income bracket would be attracted by the warm, enjoyable, and upscale surroundings and would return to the hospital or encourage others to do so. Dr. Ogunsanya was able to design a product that appealed to a target audience.

Price became a consideration, as Dr. Ogunsanya evaluated the hospital's features, advantages, and benefits. Westville Hospital was able to offer a low price point for the low- and medium-income in-patients who were treated in multi-occupancy wards. Patients who could afford it would choose to be treated in large, well-appointed private rooms. Though the entire physical facility had been upgraded, and the quality of medical delivery was the same, prices were based on a sliding scale based on what the patient was willing or able to pay.

Satisfied with his efforts to improve place, product, and price, Dr. Ogunsanya focused on promotion efforts that would tell the community about the new premium healthcare delivery services. He realized that a high-income audience would be attracted to marketing devices such as glossy magazines, brochures, and the Internet—media where he could include photos of the new premium rooms and use the type of vocabulary that a prosperous, well-educated audience would appreciate.

Jude prepared marketing messages that conveyed a sense of exclusivity in an exceptionally welcoming environment and exemplary medical care.

In less than two months, Westville Hospital began to receive an influx of patients seeking private rooms and an attractive environment. As Dr. Ogunsanya said during a meeting with his employees, "To capture an upscale audience, you must deliver an upscale experience."

## Discussion Questions

1. For 15 years, Westville Hospital had been known for quality healthcare service delivery. What might have prompted Dr. Ogunsanya to rebrand the hospital to attract an upscale audience? Was this change justifiable from a financial perspective? Why and why not?
2. Imagine that Dr. Ogunsanya's efforts had not yielded positive results, either financial or to raise the hospital's image in the community. Would his efforts to improve place, product, price, and promotion have been a waste of money? Did he need to work with Jude to create a new marketing campaign, or make adjustments to product and price in order to maintain the hospital's valued reputation while maintaining a healthy budget?

## References

Albert, N., Merunka, D., & Valette-Florence, P. (2008). When consumers love their brands: Exploring the concept and its dimensions. *Journal of Business Research, 61*(10), 1062–1075.

Anderson, J. C., & Narus, J. A. (2003). Selectively pursuing more of your customer's business. *MIT Sloan Management Review, 44*(3), 42–49.

Bonoma, T. V., & Shapiro, B. P. (1984). Evaluating market segmentation approaches. *Industrial Marketing Management, 13*(4), 257–268.

Brooksbank, R. (1994). The anatomy of marketing positioning strategy. *Marketing Intelligence & Planning, 12*(4), 10–14.

Chahal, H., & Bala, M. (2012). Significant components of service brand equity in healthcare sector. *International Journal of Health Care Quality Assurance, 25*(4), 343–362.

Christensen, C. M., Anthony, S. D., Berstell, G., & Nitterhouse, D. (2007). Finding the right job for your product. *MIT Sloan Management Review, 48*(3), 38–47.

D'Aveni, R. A. (2007). Mapping your competitive position. *Harvard Business Review, 85*(11), 110.

Davidson, S. (2001). Seizing your competitive advantage. *America's Community Banker, 10*(8), 32–33.

Dibb, S., & Simkin, L. (1997). A program for implementing market segmentation. *Journal of Business & Industrial Marketing, 12*(1), 51–65.

Dibb, S., Stern, P., & Wensley, R. (2002). Academic views on market segmentation. *Marketing Intelligence and Planning, 20,* 113–119.

Engel, J. F., Fiorillo, H. F., & Cayley, M. A. (1972). *Market segmentation: Concepts and applications.* New York, NY: Holt, Rineholt and Winston.

Fischer, S. (2014). Hospital positioning and integrated hospital marketing communications: State-of-the-art review, conceptual framework, and research agenda. *Journal of Nonprofit & Public Sector Marketing, 26*(1), 1–34.

Goldstein, S. M., Ward, P. T., Leong, G. K., & Butler, T. W. (2002). The effect of location, strategy, and operations technology on hospital performance. *Journal of Operations Management, 20*(1), 63–75.

Hlavacka, S., Bacharova, L., Rusnakova, V., & Wagner, R. (2001). Performance implications of Porter's generic strategies in Slovak hospitals. *Journal of Management in Medicine, 15*(1), 44–66.

Hopps, J. (n.d.). Target market selection segmentation and positioning. *Demand Metrics Blog.* Retrieved from https://blog.demandmetric.com/2008/08/06/target-market-selection-segmentation-and-positioning

Keller, K. L. (2008). *Best practice cases in branding: Lessons from the world's strongest brands.* Upper Saddle River, NJ: Pearson.

Kemp, E., Jillapalli, R., & Becerra, E. (2014). Healthcare branding: Developing emotionally based consumer brand relationships. *Journal of Services Marketing, 28*(2), 126–137.

Kim, K. H., Kim, K. S., Kim, D. Y., Kim, J. H., & Kang, S. H. (2008). Brand equity in hospital marketing. *Journal of Business Research, 61*(1), 75–82.

Kotler, P., & Keller, K. L. (2005). *Marketing management.* Harlow, England: Prentice-Hall.

Kotler, P., & Keller, K. L. (2006). *Identifying market segments and targets: Marketing management* (12th ed.). Singapore: Pearson Education Singapore.

Markgraf, B. (n.d.). How is competitive advantage used in focus strategy? Retrieved from http://smallbusiness.chron.com/competitive-advantage -used-focus-strategy-51750.html

McDonald, M., & Dunbar, I. (2004). *Marketing segmentation.* Oxford, England: Butterworth-Heinemann.

McGovern, G., & Moon, Y. (2007). Companies and the customers who hate them. *Harvard Business Review, 85*(6), 78–84.

Moschis, G., & Friend, S. (2008). Segmenting the preferences & usage patterns of the mature consumer health care market. *International Journal of Pharmaceutical and Healthcare Marketing, 2*(1), 7–21.

Porter, M. (1987, May/June). From competitive advantage to corporate strategy. *Harvard Business Review.* Retrieved from https://hbr.org/1987/05/ from-competitive-advantage-to-corporate-strategy

Porter, M. E. (1980). *Competitive strategy: Techniques for analyzing industries' competitors.* New York, NY: The Free Press.

Porter, M. E. (1985). *Competitive advantage: Creating and sustaining superior performance.* New York, NY: Free Press.

Ross, C. K., Steward, C. A., & Sinacore, J. M. (1993). The importance of patient preferences in the measurement of health care satisfaction. *Medical Care, 31*(12), 1138–1149.

Smith, D. C., & Park, C. W. (1992). The effects of brand extensions on market share and advertising efficiency. *Journal of Marketing Research, 29*(3), 296–313.

Simkin, L. (2008). Achieving market segmentation from B2B sectorisation. *Journal of Business & Industrial Marketing, 23*(7), 464–474.

Skinner, N. (2017, September 19). Technology's vital role in healthcare and society. Retrieved from https://www.himss.org/news/technology-s-vital -role-healthcare-and-society-national-health-it-week

Thompson, A. A., Strickland, A. J., Gamble, J. E., & Zeng'an G. (2008). *Crafting and executing strategy: The quest for competitive advantage: Concepts and cases* (19th ed.). New York, NY: McGraw-Hill Education.

Vandermerwe, S. (2004). Achieving deep customer focus. *MIT Sloan Management Review, 45*(3), 26–34.

Weinstein, A. (2004). *Handbook of market segmentation: Strategic targeting for business and technology firms.* New York, NY: Haworth.

Wu, C.-C. (2011). The impact of hospital brand image on service quality, patient satisfaction and loyalty. *African Journal of Business Management, 5*(12), 4873–4882.

# 10

## *Balancing Healthcare Service Demand and Capacity*

## Chapter Outline

- Introduction
- Fluctuations in Demand and Healthcare Service Productivity
- Demand and Capacity of a Healthcare Service Organization
- Managing Demand Levels and Waiting Times
- Inventory Holding
- Inventory Models
- Managing Perceptions of Waiting Time
- Conclusion
- Review Questions
- Mini Case Study With Discussion Questions
- References

*Marketing in Healthcare-Related Industries*, pages 227–243
Copyright © 2020 by Information Age Publishing
All rights of reproduction in any form reserved.

## Chapter Outcome

By the end of this chapter, the reader will be able to

- explain how fluctuations in demand threaten service productivity,
- explain the idea that "many service organizations are capacity-constrained,"
- discuss the patterns and determinations of demand,
- explain how demand levels can be managed,
- discuss inventory demand through waiting lines and reservations,
- explain how to minimize perceptions of waiting time, and
- explain how to create an effective reservations system.

## Introduction

The ability of a health service firm to be a significant force in the industry in which it operates, is dependent on its ability to manage demand and capacity effectively. The management of demand and capacity in the service context allows firms to meet customer requirements in an effective and efficient manner, that is, minimizing resources and time. For instance, a business-oriented reservation system has to apply the current technology to allow hoteliers to have a competitive advantage over their competitors and to maintain their position at the forefront of emerging trends in the environment. A modern reservation system must not only be about registering clinical bookings, for example, instead, it must be able to either propose or connect easily to extra services. The main things to look out for in a reservation system is the capacity to quickly, easily, and effectively manage online rate and inventory distribution across all channels. Coordinating the needed activities, however, involves some complexity which if not properly managed can increase administration lapses and a greater probability of errors in data inputs.

It is the desire of prudent health service firms to use available resources in the best manner to satisfy customers at the right time, hence, the need for demand and capacity management. This chapter, therefore, discusses demand fluctuations and service productivity, managing demand levels, and minimizing perceptions of waiting time, among others.

## Fluctuations in Demand and Healthcare Service Productivity

Unlike goods and physical products, health services cannot be easily stockpiled (Kotler, 2003), and this is a challenge for the health service industry when it comes to managing demand. The objective in the health service sector is to use available resources such as staff, equipment, and facilities as productively as possible. In this instance, there is a need to introduce what is termed the health service decision framework. When making decisions on matching demand and capacity, the following questions must be answered: What sort of business is this? Therefore, in the service processes, what can be utilized in operation? Who is defined as the target market, and how should the relationship? What are the core and supplementary elements of service? How should charges be priced (price and other outlays)? How should information be communicated to customers?

In the last decade, the health service sector has witnessed a major boost in the world economy, and its importance has been well-established. For example, the uses of services and products that are physical in nature have been seen as a major integration solution to customers. In recent times, health service provision has been understood to be a value-addition, an "add-on" for goods that are tangible. Contrarily, the service-dominant logic which is emerging in the business domain sees goods as mere appliances for service delivery. This chapter explores how fluctuation in demand threatens health service productivity.

In healthcare, value co-creation is an emerging and effective way for physicians and patients to ameliorate health outcomes, and it is contingent on the relationship among stakeholders: patients, patients' families, caregivers, and healthcare organizations (Anderson, Rayburn, & Sierra, 2019). An understanding of consumer-value co-creation can help healthcare organizations adopt appropriate strategies and practices which will recognize consumers as partners in the development and delivery of innovative healthcare products and services (Nambisan & Nambisan, 2009). Therefore, a health service includes at least two partners: a service provider applying skills and a customer that assimilates the applied know-hows with other resources; therefore, value is always co-created (Spohrer, Maglio, Bailey, & Gruhl, 2007). Service productivity, generally, is

> a function of (1) how effectively input resources into the service (production) process are transformed to outputs in the form of services (internal efficiency), (2) how well the quality of the service process and its outcome is perceived (external efficiency or effectiveness) and (3) how effectively the capacity of the service process is utilized (capacity efficiency). (Grönroos & Ojasalo, 2004, p. 414)

According to Lovelock, Wirtz, and Chew (2009), health service productivity can take several forms in services, which include the following:

- physical facilities designed to contain customers;
- physical facilities designed for storing or processing goods;

- physical equipment used to process people, possessions, or information;
- labor; and
- infrastructure.

Also, according to them, there are four conditions possibly faced by service productivity, and they are as follows:

- excess demand (high demand relative to capacity at a given time);
- demand exceeds desired capacity (no one is turned away—the point beyond which service quality declines as more customers are serviced);
- demand and supply are well-balanced at desired capacity (staff and facilities are busy without being overworked and customers receive good service without delay); and
- excess capacity relative to demand at a given time with underutilized resources and low productivity).

Lovelock et al. (2009), state in relation to the second point that an oscillation in demand affects service productivity negatively. In relation to the forms of service productivity, an increase in demand will lead to their decline. With service productivity in the form of a physical facility designed to contain customers, an increase in demand will decline its effectiveness. For instance, the constant use of public transport will, due to its high patronage over time, experience a reduction in its effectiveness and may eventually break down. Health service productivity in the form of physical facilities designed to store and process goods or products will decline with an increase in demand. For example, the endless use of a combined harvester machine to harvest rice to meet the increasing demand of consumers will eventually break the machine down. The effectiveness of the combined harvester reduces first, and further constant use of it breaks it down.

Health service productivity in labor also decays with an increase in demand. According to *The Business Dictionary* (n.d.), labor is referred to as "the aggregate of human physical and mental efforts in the creation of goods and services." Briefly, labor has to do with human effort, and in the healthcare sector, it encompasses professionals like laboratory technologists, doctors, nurses, and pharmacists, to name a few. To the extent that demand for health services is very high in most emerging economies of the world, health service labor is often compelled to put in extra hours to meet the high health service demand. Continual production to meet the high health demand could lead to a reduction in the energy used by the health labor force, which in turn affects the level of productivity.

Infrastructure, as a form of service productivity, is also diminished as a result of fluctuations in demand. According to *The Business Dictionary* (n.d), infrastructure refers to "the relatively permanent and foundational capital investment of a country, firm, or project that underlies and makes possible all its economic activity." For example, an auditorium built for a city with a capacity of 10,000 people and theoretically to be used once a week, is instead being used 3 times a week and always with full seating capacity. Without proper care and management, the auditorium will lose its quality of service. To conclude, Lovelock et al. (2009) gave two primary tactics to address the problem of fluctuating demand which are:

- altering the level of capacity to meet demand, which has to do with the consideration of productive capacity and how it can vary on an incremental basis; and
- managing level of demand by using marketing strategies to even out peaks and fill in gaps.

As a result of the nature and characteristics of a health service, most health organizations in developing nations are capacity constrained. The capacity of a health institution is the ability of the institution to meet demand and the extent to which it can do it. In terms of production of goods, it can easily be expanded or contracted. However, when it relates to service delivery, it becomes very difficult as a result of four main challenges: time, labor, equipment, and facilities.

Health capacity management is the ability to bring equilibrium to the demand from customers, and also the ability of the service delivery system to satisfy these demands. This first places emphasis on understanding the nature of demand by projecting (Lovelock, 1984) and second, the choices for managing capacity to meet the likely demand. Sasser (1976, as cited in Armistead & Clark, 1991) suggests two basic plans for capacity in services, namely *level* and *chase*, while the former is applicable where capacity is limited, and hence, the focus is on inducing demand to be in line with capacity. The latter strategy occurs when supply can be changed in line with demand. This implies that an operations manager must understand the composition of their capacity, the degree to which it can be changed, the speed of reaction, and the costs involved (Armistead & Clark, 1991). This book acknowledges this and discusses it in detail.

Defining services as intangible products signifies that intangible products can array from electric service to education, to financial services, and from healthcare to hospitality, and then to sports. One of the more commonly used definitions of service is, "An act or performance offered by one party to another. Although the process may be tied to a physical product, the performance is essentially intangible and does not result in ownership of any of the factors of production" (Lovelock, 2000, p. 3). Pine and Gilmore (1999) also defined services as "intangible actions tailored to the individual request of known clients" (p. 8). Bowen and Ford (2002) suggest that an intangible service includes all the fundamentals that come together to create an unforgettable knowledge for a customer at a point in time. These elements include an intangible or tangible service product and other systems that permit the delivery of the service experience to the customer.

Unlike tangible products, health services rendered by most health service organizations cannot be inventoried because of their perishable nature. Bowen and Ford (2002) also claim that services cannot be stored because there is nothing to store; thus, they are perishable. Since services cannot be stored, inventions obviously cannot start until the customer demands them. Therefore, production is often concurrent with consumption. To that end, Sasser (1976) notes that because services typically involve simultaneous production and consumption, it will be hard to inventory intangible products to match capacity with demand. The doubt of demand creates problems for service organizations as to how, when, and where to increase their service capacity, since these intangible products cannot be reserved for future use.

Marketing intangible products creates some exclusive challenges for managers. A survey conducted by Zeithaml, Parasuraman, and Berry (1985), showed that service managers rated *fluctuating service demand* as their greatest test. Bowen and Ford (2002) also note that since there is no physical inventory, demand cannot be smoothed through inventories. For instance, few rooms available in a hotel resort during normal days cannot be inventoried or warehoused for the holiday periods, because the demand for rooms will surpass the capacity of the hotel resort during the holiday period. Kotler, Bowen, and Makens (1999) also note that since services cannot be inventoried, management of demand is more sensitive to time. Because of this, services often use promotions and lower prices to increase demand during relaxed periods (Sasser, 1976).

However, Bowen and Ford (2002) argue that if there is too much capacity, then the sluggish capacity costs will likely make the firm more uncompetitive than organizations that have been more successful in matching their capacity and demand. If there is not enough capacity to meet demand, the firm runs the risk of losing customers. Klassen and Rohlender (2001) point out that the ambiguity of demand, which can fluctuate on an hour-by-hour basis, makes managing capacity and demand in services difficult. They went on to suggest that service organizations must find ways to balance capacity with demand without the benefit of the manufacturers' physical inventory buffer or the risk of losing customers who refuse to wait for service.

According to Sasser (1976), increasing customer input can also increase capacity. However, customer participation can create uncertainty in a number of ways. Customers may not appreciate the service offering or their role in obtaining the service experience. When this happens, the employee has to spend more time with the customer, often triggering delays for other customers. The process of rendering services may be perceived as arduous by some customers as the time required in the service experience may not be expected standard and, thus, negatively affects the service organization's ability to match capacity and demand (Booms & Bitner, 1981).

Heskett, Sasser, and Hart (1990) note the importance of keeping demand as close to the optimal capacity level as possible. The authors, however, indicate that "this does not imply a target of 100 percent capacity exploitation, a major factor of success in many services is the degree to which accessible capacity is utilized" (1990, p. 137). They further state that capacity utilization varies inversely with some factors. One of these factors includes the degree to which a service capacity is fixed. According to Klassen and Rohleder (2001), the reason why this occurs is that the more capacity is fixed, the less flexibility a service has to match demand. For instance, assuming a bank resolves to have a fixed number of 10 tellers serving its customers without being allowed to do any other task, then the bank will suffer lower teller utilization at less busy times than if it had the tractability to vary the number of tellers and tasks they perform by adjustment of cost. Proper inventory management enables organizations to minimize cost and maximize profit.

## Demand and Capacity of a Healthcare Service Organization

Healthcare demand is not a factor that can be easily controlled since it changes at a given time, in any situation and period. Therefore, it is important to understand its patterns and determinants in order to come to terms with how to manage it. To do this, it is important that questions, such as "Does demand trigger some predictable cycle, and if so, what are the underlying causes of cyclical variations (employment, billing and tax payment, wage/salary, school hours, vacations, climate, public/religious holidays, natural—coastal tides)?"; "Do demand levels seem to change haphazardly (due to weather, health issues—heart attacks and births—accidents, criminal activities)?"; and "Can demand over time be disaggregated by market?"

Demand can sometimes behave in a chance pattern and irregular manner. The three types of demand behavior are the trend, the cycle, and the seasonal patterns. A trend is a gradual, long term up and down movement of demand. Trends are often the starting points for developing forecast. Random variations can be considered to be activities which are not predictable and therefore, follow no particular pattern. To manage fluctuation demand in a service business, it is important to have a rich understanding of demand patterns, reasons for variation, and the market segments that encompass demand at different points in time (Chetty & Coetzee, 2010).

The following are, therefore, key to understanding demand patterns and the determination of demand: the first is plotting demand patterns. According to Chetty and Coetzee (2010), the firm should chart the levels of demand over the germane time periods. The firm that creates very good relationships with its customers can do this very quickly. The second is predictable cycles. When the graphical pattern of demand level is considered, the following questions are asked: Is there a clear cycle daily (variations in hours)? Weekly (variations occur by day) or monthly (variations occur by weeks)? If there is a predictable cycle, what are the roots? This can assist a service provider in dealing with the customers more efficiently. The third is the random demand vacillations. At times, the patterns of demand may not be vibrant, where there is no apparent predictable cycle. Yet in this case, causes can be recognized. For instance, day-to-day changes in the weather may affect the use of a recreational facility, and although the weather cannot be predicted far in advance (Chetty & Coetzee, 2010), it may be possible to understand demand a day or two ahead.

Health linked issues cannot be predicted. Coincidences, such as heart attacks or other sudden emergencies all increase demand for hospital services, but the level of demand cannot be normally determined in advance. Natural disasters such as floods, fires, and hurricanes can farcically increase the demand for such services as insurance, telecommunication, and healthcare. If an organization has detailed records on customer activities, it may be able to disaggregate demand by market segmentation, revealing patterns within patterns.

## Managing Demand Levels and Waiting Times

According to Croxton, Lambert, García-Dastugue, and Rogers (2002), "Demand management is the supply chain management process that balances the customers' requirements with the capabilities of the supply chain" (p. 51). It relates to forecasting and synchronizing the strategic processes of a firm for the purpose of designing an efficient operational system for matching supply and demand. This can be at macro levels as in economics and at micro levels within individual organizations. For example, at macro levels, a government may sway interest rates in order to adjust financial demand. This study discusses how demand levels can be managed.

Philip Kotler notes that first, demand management is the duty of the marketing organization (as sales are a subset of marketing). Second, demand "forecast" is an outcome of planned marketing efforts. The purpose of these planned marketing efforts should go beyond stimulating demand to influencing demand so that the objectives of the organization will be achieved (Kotler, 2000).

Operations managers in a health service organization will either thrive or flop in the process of balancing quality of service and resource management, in terms of resource productivity, depending on their skills and expertise. Chase practices are applicable when customers will not be queueing to be attended to, and there is an urgent need to ensure the process commences and that it is taken to a reasonable stage for customer satisfaction. The concept of a coping strategy for managing a health service asset has a particular link to service recovery (Hart, Heskett, & Sasser, 1990). It appears, however, that managing coping appears to be a less practiced concept by practitioners than service recovery. Armstead (1990), has suggested that having an understanding of the service operations task is instrumental for translating service strategy into a service delivery concept which is capable of achieving the goals of the strategy.

Larsson and Bowen (1989) propose a model that addresses the aspect of uncertainty in demand, first, in the mix of services required and second, in the nature of demand related to customers' willingness to participate. Demand control describes the management of demand and supply in instances where there is an unexpected change in demand or a sudden demand. Changes in demand occur when near-term demand exceeds supply or when the actual orders are less than expected. Changes in demand, if not handled properly, can lead to reactive decisions, which can, in turn, have a negative effect on the workload of employees, costs, and the ability of the firm to satisfy customers. To mitigate the effects of changes in demand calls for demand controls. It creates synchronization across the different functions of the business such as sales, demand planning, and supply planning. An advantage of demand control is that analysis of demand is done at regular intervals like daily or weekly, unlike the typical monthly demand or supply planning reviews. Frequent analyses of demand allow organizations to respond quickly as well as be proactive in handling possible imbalances in demand and supply (Croxton et al., 2002; Fahrioglu & Alvarado, 2000).

Customers often have to pause during the process of attaining and consuming products and services. The waiting practices are typically considered to have negative influence on customers' overall satisfaction with the products and services (Kumar, Kalwani, & Dada, 1997; Davis & Heineke, 1998), so the importance of proper management of customers' waiting time is of significant interest to most organizations (Au, 2009; Kumar et al., 1997; Larson, 1987; Peter & Peppiatt, 1996; Taylor, 1994; ). Managers should not only focus on reducing actual waiting times but also to explore new ways of improving customer satisfaction with a given waiting time. Many firms institute a variation of programs to augment customer waiting experience.

An important initiative that many health services firms have undertaken for managing customers' waiting time is the institution of waiting-time guarantees (Allon & Federgruen, 2008; Babad, Dada, & Saharia, 1996; Kumar et al., 1997; So & Song, 1998 ). Numerous service industries use waiting time standards as a clearly advertised competitive tool. For instance, banks such as Wells Fargo award $5 when a customer waits more than 5 minutes in line (Allon & Federgruen, 2008).

Research on customer waiting time has customarily been the domain of the queuing theory. Queues occur because the environment is uncertain; whenever the demand for service exceeds the ability to provide service, a queue forms. A major dissimilarity classifies queues according to the number of servers and the distributions that characterize the arrival rates of customers (or their inter-arrival times) and the service times.

Every current operations management textbook contains a chapter with a title like "Inventory Management" (Heizer & Render, 2006) or "Inventory Planning and Control" (Slack, Chambers & Johnston, 2004). The content refers to the ongoing provision of standard items with free demand, where some speculative quantity should always be on hand. Businesses hold these stocks for various reasons, including protection against general shortages or potential problems with suppliers, or, because unit price rises may be imminent. Nevertheless, the literature focuses on stock refill policies. Typically, the resultant inventories enable firms to perform a service thriftily, without the beneficiaries suffering any untoward delays. The inventory demand can be determined through waiting lines and reservation systems.

The theory's building block is the economic order quantity (EOQ) model, which divulges the optimum amount Q to reorder for an individual item. Several (possible) operating systems are available for monitoring stock levels and initiating fresh orders. Moreover, different items should not be treated equally, since a certain minority will be highly influential. The literature proffers advice on these practical matters but tends to be inconsistent, muddled, and even illogical at times. Moreover, the EOQ model is myopic because it only considers the purchasing side, taking no direct account of how the supplier organizes, plans, and executes the processing, picking, and transportation of various customers' orders.

Supply chain management (SCM) covers more than one site and is a "hot topic" in operations management. It is a natural leeway of the materials that necessities planning (MNP) and enterprise resources planning (ERP) systems common in manufacturing applications, whereby, all dependent demands falling in any specific time period can be designed precisely. The necessary purchasing and production activities are scheduled accordingly and linked to the provision of matching resources. To date, neither SCM's emergence exerted minimal influence on stock control theory, nor the underlying "just-in-time" (JIT) philosophy has had a noticeable impact, despite comments that process improvements are more fruitful than tinkering with mathematical models (Knod & Schonberger, 2001). Nissan's U.K. supplier pick-up routes, or "milk rounds," are a prime example (Wickens, 1998). Relying on the milk rounds ideology, Nissan U.K. uses a central hub or transshipment center for reporting and consolidating inbound delivery.

## Inventory Holding

For a health organization, it becomes important to hold inventory for the following reason:

- Inventory holding ensures that operation delays do not impact delivery to customers.
- It also ensures that the organization meets full demand or fluctuations in demand.
- It ensures that the productions of the company are flexible.
- It ensures that supplier delays do not affect the working of the company.

Considering the above inventory holding objectives, the next step for the health company is to make inventory-related decisions. Inventory decision involves two major deliberations, first, is quantity of the raw material needed for orders, and second, the timing for placing those orders.

## Inventory Models

Inventory management can be explained by using two basic models: the independent demand inventory model and the dependent demand inventory model (Urban, 2005).

1. The *independent demand inventory model* describes how the demand for some raw materials used by a firm is not reliant on the demand for another item. It relates to the demand for finished goods.
2. The *dependent demand inventory model* relates to the demand for raw materials which are integral parts of production and form an important part of material resource planning. For example, demand for raw materials can be established as the basis of demand for finished products.

## Managing Perceptions of Waiting Time

When health service customers find it difficult to get information, they develop high perceptions and fear of waiting times. In the marketing and consumer research literature, several studies have examined waiting times for services within the contexts of hospitals, banks, and other service industries (e.g., Hui & Tse, 1996; Katz, Larson, & Larson, 1991; Pruyn & Smidts, 1999). Other studies have explored the waiting-time fillers on consumer perceptions and evaluations of waiting times (e.g., Katzet et al., 1991; Pruyn & Smidts, 1998; Taylor, 1994; Tom, Burns, & Zeng, 1997). The latter is based on the idea of changing waiting time into experienced time by "entertaining, enlightening, and engaging" the consumer (Katz et al., 1991).

Waiting in a queue for a long time for a health service is a situation every customer wants to avoid. Waiting in queues is not new to most consumers of the post office, grocery shops, airports, mobile phone shops, or high street retail shops as they encounter it daily. Queuing has cost implications on both the customers and companies. Therefore, it is now the modern marketing practices for businesses and academics to conduct a wide array of research and undertake insight analytics geared towards mitigating the negative effects of queuing on the customer's perceived experience (Tamuno, 2013).

Mainster (1985), a renowned scholar in the area of psychology of waiting times, developed a formula on the topic, $S = P - E$. According to the author, the $S$ represents satisfaction, $P$ stands for perception, and $E$ signifies expectation. The author further notes $S$ is achieved when a customer's $P$ of the service received surpasses his or her expectations. Related to waiting lines, customers often feel excited when they spend less time than anticipated in waiting to receive a service.

A research conducted by Jones and Peppiatt (1996) on consumer perception of waiting times in different service queues reveals that businesses often work on reducing the actual time the customer spends waiting as a measure to deal with waiting time rather than to influence the perception these customers hold about the waiting times. They add that there is a gap between a customer's perception of the waiting time and the actual waiting time, which firms must deal with. In his work which which examines the psychology of waiting times, Mainster (1984) asserts that occupied time feels shorter than unoccupied time. Companies are introducing solutions via technological products on the shop floor or service points in order to entertain and engage customers while they wait. There are a number of methods and products that can assist a company in mitigating the perceived waiting times of customers. The first strategy is television entertainment. This is a common product used by many businesses, as Thomke (2003) indicates that customers' waiting time decreased from 32% to 26% in bank branches which had televisions in their lobbies. Axis Satellite, a leading television entertainment provider, adds that although customers' waiting time can negatively affect their willingness to spend, providing television entertainment can reduce a customer's perceived waiting time and spur their willingness to spend (Tamuno, 2013).

Finally, the use of fragrance is a very important aspect of the waiting time experience, which tends to be ignored by most businesses. The fragrance-laden shop floor environment motivates some people to go window shopping in perfume shops. It is very important that a soothing and inspiring environment is created because when customers enjoy and appreciate the service environment, they are more likely to return and even recommend the organization to others. In most progressive hospitals the world over, healthcare managers are investing heavily in removing the usual smells associated with medicines and cleaning detergents mostly associated with hospital service delivery. The pleasant fragrances created as a result are meant to enhance the hospital attendance experience.

## Conclusion

This chapter recognizes the value of being able to manage demand and capacity effectively. As with all businesses, it is essential for organizations to be prudent and use available resources in the best manner to satisfy customers at the right time. Hence, the need for demand and capacity management. This chapter, therefore, discusses demand fluctuations and service productivity, managing demand levels, and minimizing perceptions of waiting time, among others.

While recognizing the contribution of healthcare services in the world's economic boom, practitioners need to be aware of the fluctuation in demand and healthcare service productivity. Measures should be put in place to manage it effectively; this includes inventory holding, managing staff and other stakeholders, even to the extent of managing customers' waiting time. This ensures that resources are well managed and not drained unnecessarily, especially for those health organizations that solely receive their funds from the government, which can be limited.

## Review Questions

1. Explain how fluctuations in demand threaten service productivity.
2. Explain the idea that "many service organizations are capacity-constrained."
3. Discuss the need for healthcare to manage their limited resources.

### MINI CASE STUDY: HANDLING WAITING TIME

Sylvester Gomnah suddenly fell seriously ill with chest pains and nausea, and Kuma, his roommate, rushed him to Seth District Hospital in Nairobi, Kenya. On arrival, they were directed to a waiting room where a nurse recorded Sylvester's symptoms and then left them there. Thirty minutes passed, and they were yet to see the doctor. Kuma was becoming increasingly anxious about his friend's pain, and he got the attention of a nurse, Selina. She apologized for the delay, explaining that the doctor was attending to an emergency case but should be available in 10 minutes or so. While she was talking to them, Selina saw that Sylvester was shivering and beginning to gasp for breath. She quickly found a wheelchair and got him to a treatment room, helped him onto the bed, took his vital signs, and fixed some blankets to calm the situation while they waited. Kuma sat beside the bed and spoke quietly to Sylvester, watching as his friend eventually calmed down and fell into a troubled sleep. Selina returned and found that Sylvester was no longer running a dangerously high temperature. Kuma was happy that Selina had taken charge of the situation and helped his friend before his friend's condition worsened. Kuma was impressed by the outstanding service rendered by Selina.

After about an hour, Sylvester woke up and said he was very thirsty. Immediately, Kuma found a water dispenser nearby and encouraged his friend to drink slowly. The doctor arrived then and apologized, explaining the cause of the delay just as Selina had described earlier. The doctor examined Sylvester, ordered some blood tests, and offered a diagnosis of food poisoning. He was given a prescription and told that he would soon feel better. Thankful and feeling much better, Sylvester and Kuma left the hospital. Both were very impressed with the treatment Sylvester had received, and both were happy to recommend Seth District Hospital to others, primarily because of the way the nurse, Selina, had handled the situation while they waited to see the doctor.

## Discussion Questions

1. If Selina had not acted the way she did, in this case, Kuma's perception of Seth District Hospital would likely have been quite negative. Describe the implications this negative impression would have had on the hospital's marketing strategy. When does word-of-mouth become more influential than a well-planned marketing campaign? When does it not?
2. Explain how Seth District Hospital might have offered the needed training and guidance that empowered Selina to take Sylvester into the treatment room. How could her actions be included in an operational procedure that would assure the public of excellent treatment?

# References

Allon, G., & Federgruen, A. (2008). Service competition with general queuing facilities. *Operations Research, 56*(4), 827–849.

Armistead, C. G. (1990). Service operations strategy: Framework for matching the service operations task and the service delivery system. *International Journal of Service Industry Management, 1*(2).

Armistead, C., & Clark G. (1991). *Capacity management in services and the influence on quality and productivity performance.* Retrieved from https://dspace.lib .cranfield.ac.uk/bitstream/handle/1826/333/SWP5691.pdf?sequence=2

Anderson, S., Rayburn, S. W., & Sierra, J. J. (2019). Future thinking: The role of marketing in healthcare. *European Journal of Marketing, 53*(8), 1521–1545. https://doi.org/10.1108/EJM-10-2017-0779

Babad, Y., Dada, M., & Saharia, A. (1996). An appointment-based service center with guaranteed service. *European Journal of Operational Research, 89*(2), 246–258.

Booms, B. H., & Bitner, M. J. (1981). Marketing strategies and organization structures for service firms. *Marketing of Services, 25*(3), 47–52.

Bowen, J., & Ford, R. C. (2002). Managing service organizations: Does having a "thing" make a difference? *Journal of Management, 28*(3), 447–469.

Chetty, J., & Coetzee, M. (2010). Towards an information security framework for service-oriented architect. In *2010 Information Security for South Africa* (pp. 1–8). IEEE. Retrieved from https://doi.org/10.1109/issa.2010 .5588272

Croxton, K. L., Lambert, D. M., García-Dastugue, S. J., & Rogers, D. S. (2002). The demand management process. *The International Journal of Logistics Management, 13*(2), 51–66.

Davis, M., & Heineke, J. (1998). How disconfirmation, perception and actual waiting times impact customer satisfaction. *International Journal of Service Industry Management, 9*(1), 64–73.

Fahrioglu, M., & Alvarado, F. L. (2000). Designing incentive compatible contracts for effective demand management. *IEEE Transactions on power Systems, 15*(4), 1255–1260.

Grönroos, C., & Ojasalo, K. (2004). Service productivity: Towards a conceptualization of the transformation of inputs into economic results in services. *Journal of Business Research, 57*(4), 414–423.

Hart, C. W., Heskett, J. L., & Sasser Jr, W. E. (1990). The profitable art of service recovery. *Harvard Business Review, 68*(4), 148–156.

Heizer, J., & Render, B. (2006). *Operations management* (8th ed.). Upper Saddle River, NJ: Pearson Prentice-Hall.

Heskett, J. A., Sasser W. E., & Hart, C. W. (1990). *Service breakthroughs.* New York, NY: The Free Press.

Hui, M. K., & Tse, D. K. (1996). What to tell consumers in waits of different lengths: An integrative model of service evaluation. *Journal of Marketing, 60*(2), 81–90.

Jones, P., & Peppiatt, E. (1996). Managing perceptions of waiting times in service queues. *International Journal of Service Industry Management, 7*(5), 47–61.

Klassen, K. J., & Rohleder, T. R. (2001). Combining operations and marketing to manage capacity and demand in services. *Service Industries Journal, 21*(2), 1–30.

Knod, E., & Schonberger, R. (2001). *Operations management: Meeting customers' demands* (7th ed.). New York, NY: McGraw-Hill.

Kotler, P. (2000). *Marketing management. The millennium edition.* Upper Saddle River, NJ: Prentice Hall.

Kotler, P. (2003). *Marketing insights from A to Z: 80 concepts every manager needs to know.* New York, NY: John Wiley & Sons.

Kotler, P., Bowen, J., & Makens, J. (1999). *Marketing for hospitality and tourism.* Upper Saddle River, NJ: Prentice Hall.

Kumar, P., Kalwani, M. U., & Dada, M. (1997). The impact of waiting time guarantees on customers' waiting experiences. *Marketing Science, 16*(4), 295–314.

Larson, R. C. (1987). Perspectives on queues: Social justice and the psychology of queuing. *Operations Research, 35*(6), 895–905.

Larsson, R., & Bowen, D. E. (1989). Organization and customer: Managing design and coordination of services. *Academy of Management Review, 14*(2), 213–233.

Larson, R. C., Larson, B. M., & Katz, K. L. (1991). Prescription for waiting-in-line blues: Entertain, enlighten and engage. *Sloan Management Review, 32*(2), 44–55.

Lovelock, C. H. (1984). Strategies for managing demand in capacity-constrained service organizations. *The Service Industries Journal, 4*(3), 12–30.

Lovelock, C. H. (2000). *Services marketing* (4th ed.). Upper Saddle River, NJ: Prentice-Hall.

Lovelock, C., Wirtz, J., & Chew, P. (2009). *Essentials of services marketing.* Upper Saddle River NJ: Prentice-Hall.

Maister, D. H. (1984). *The psychology of waiting lines.* Boston, MA: Harvard Business School.

Nambisan, P., & Nambisan, S. (2009). Models of consumer value cocreation in health care. *Health Care Management Review, 34*(4), 344–354.

Peter, J., & Peppiatt, E. (1996). Managing perceptions of waiting times in service queues. *International Journal of Service Industry Management, 7*(5), 47–61.

Pine, B. J., & Gilmore, J. H. (1999). *The experience economy: Work is theatre & every business a stage.* Boston, MA: Harvard Business Press.

Pruyn, A., & Smidts, A. (1999). Customers' reactions to waiting: Effects of the presence of "fellow sufferers" in the waiting room. *Advances in Consumer Research, 26*(1).

Sasser, W. E. (1976). Match supply and demand in service industries. *Harvard Business Review, 54*(6), 131–140.

Slack, N., Chambers, S., & Johnston, R. (2004). *Operations management* (4th ed.). Harlow, England: Prentice-Hall.

So, K. C., & Song, J. S. (1998). Price, delivery time guarantees and capacity selection. *European Journal of Operational Research, 111*(1), 28–49.

Spohrer, J., Maglio, P. P., Bailey, J., & Gruhl, D. (2007). Steps toward a science of service systems. *Computer, 40*(1), 71–77.

Tamuno, D. (n.d.). *Managing the customer's perceived waiting time—Part 1.* Retrieved from https://customerthink.com/managing_the_customers_perceived _waiting_time_part_1/

Taylor, S. (1994). Waiting for service: The relationship between delays and the evaluation of service. *Journal of Marketing, 58*(2), 56–69.

The Business Dictionary. (n.d). Retrieved from http://www.businessdictionary. com/definition/infrastructure

Thomke, S. (2003, April). R&D comes to services: Bank of America's pathbreaking experiments. *Harvard Business Review.* Retrieved from https:// hbr.org/2003/04/rd-comes-to-services-bank-of-americas-pathbreaking -experiments

Tom, G., Burns, M., & Zeng, Y. (1997). Your life on hold: The effect of telephone waiting time on customer perception. *Journal of Direct Marketing, 11*(3), 25–31.

Urban, T. L. (2005). Inventory models with inventory-level-dependent demand: A comprehensive review and unifying theory. *European Journal of Operational Research, 162*(3), 792–804.

Wickens, P. (1998). *The ascendant organization.* Basingstoke, England: Macmillan Business.

Zeithaml, V. A., Parasuraman, A., & Berry, L. L. (1985). Problems and strategies in services marketing. *The Journal of Marketing, 49*(2), 33–46.

# 11

# Managing Relationships and Building Loyalty in Healthcare Industries

## Chapter Outline

- Introduction
- Understanding the Customer-Healthcare Firm Relationship
- Targeting the Customers
- Analyzing and Managing Customer Databases
- Building Customer Loyalty
- Customer Relationship Management in Healthcare Delivery
- Conclusion
- Review Questions
- Mini Case Study With Discussion Questions
- References

## Chapter Outcome

By the end of this chapter, the reader will be able to

- explain why targeting the right customers is essential to service delivery,
- discuss how to analyze and manage the customer base,
- explain how to build customer loyalty, and
- discuss the customer relationship management system in delivering healthcare service.

## Introduction

There is a critical goal of every healthcare organization and that is to serve its customers better (Woo, Bae, & Park, 2016). To be able to achieve this goal, healthcare firms must understand that customers remain essential to them. Without their satisfaction being met, healthcare firms do not have any purpose of existing. In practice, this means that employees within every firm need to portray good behavior, not only to satisfy customers with services rendered, but also to develop a long-lasting relationship and build customer loyalty. Customer loyalty has many benefits to a healthcare organization. They include positive word-of-mouth marketing, justified price premiums, and lower employee turnover as well as reduced costs of training new employees, all resulting in higher firm profits. Firms should have knowledge about their customers; meaning, they should appreciate their existence as well as their impending customers' needs and preferences (Lee, Naylor, & Chen, 2011).

Healthcare firms should generally strive to gain an understanding of what their customers want, to build connections. By doing this, healthcare companies can collect information on how customers spend money, find out what customers want, and subsequently make predictions on what customers may demand. Thus, according to Gibbert, Leibold, and Probst (2002), healthcare enterprises ought to cautiously spot, relate with, as well as generate discourses with their customers, to attain information about them, to be able to offer tailored services and sustain continuing connections in a reliable long-term relationship. According to Mithas, Krishnan, and Fornell (2005), by having good relations with its customers, a healthcare enterprise will be able to gain information about their customers. This is associated with gaining information from customers about merchandise or amenities that can accommodate orientations to cater to these customers; additionally, this practice becomes useful for customers' contentment, customers' loyalty, and staff's output.

To build good customer relationships and in turn, build loyalty, a healthcare organization must first understand what constitutes customer loyalty. That is, the healthcare organization should clearly define the exact needs of potential and existing customers and what can be accomplished in line with the organization's tactical objectives. Then, the organization should actually put practices in place to track customers' loyalty with various performance indicators, such as customer satisfaction and customer complaints, and engage customers with the organization in an effort to increase the results on these performance indicators. Lastly, the healthcare organization has to act on the outcomes of the performance indicators to influence the attitude of customers positively.

## Understanding the Customer-Healthcare Firm Relationship

Health service marketing concerns how firms connect well interactively with customers (Reibstein, Day, & Wind, 2009). Numerous healthcare enterprises spend a sizeable amount of money on relationship marketing (RM)—the process of developing cooperative and collaborative relationships with customers and other market actors (Sheth & Parvatiyar, 1995), in order to achieve a closer affiliation with their customers, with the belief that the efforts will achieve positive monetary results. Hospitals can overcome the challenges of competitive threat by engaging in relationship marketing activities and developing cooperative relationships with customers, suppliers, and other healthcare providers (Naidu, Parvatiyar, Sheth, & Westgate, 1999). However, other customers remain unresponsive or antagonistic to an enterprise relations-building effort according to Godfrey, Seiders, and Voss (2011). Enterprises, however, need to apportion their means to their customers who are predicted to be amenable to relationship marketing (Palmatier, 2008). According to Keller and Lehmann (2006), "Healthcare service marketers should delve into the appropriate ways, customer preferred affiliation can be affirmed if customers still desire close relationships with companies, as well as the ways in which a desired customer relationship can be cultivated by the company through marketing activities" (p. 742).

The interdependence theory suggests that having a closer affirmation with customers whereby the two parties, (i.e., the healthcare customer and the healthcare provider) have a recurrent and solid influence on each other in various situations is a desirable situation for any forward-looking healthcare organization.

Health service marketers should know what the customers needs are, so that their organizations can meet the demands, in order to encourage repeat business. This helps to enhance and intensify the customers and the firm interactions for a longer time, thereby tightening the bond between them, and also sustain a good relationship leading to the commitment between both parties. Dagger, Danaher, and Gibbs (2009) note that customers who are more interactive with firms tend to build stronger relationships. One way of interacting with a healthcare institution that helps to meet the understanding of the client and firm bond is operational marketing. Operational marketing involves the interchange of what both the healthcare customer and service provider will gain at the end. A customer database is another form of operational marketing that can be a contributor to building a good customer-firm relationship. Through the database, the emphasis is still on marketing operation, and healthcare marketers depend on patient information and records to support their continued rapport with clients.

One other way an enterprise can build a good connection with its clients is to practice relationship marketing. Relationship marketing occurs when a particular healthcare firm is able to extend a long-lasting bond between them and their clients. Copulsky and Wolf (1990) contend that relationship building with customers is necessary, considering the cost involved in attaining a new customer and the customer's lifetime-value to a hospital; it could, for instance, benefit the hospital by keeping the customer for 50 years.

## Targeting the Customers

Acquiring and retaining customers should be an important consideration of every health service firm. In this regard, there is the need for health service firms to recruit the right customers so that they can provide the needed services efficiently, in order to enhance their customer's satisfaction and improve their loyalty levels. Moreover, aside the required clients' services, there is a need for health firms to also devise other well-supported strategies targeted at making consumers prefer their brands. Examples of these strategies include giving of rewards and facilitating executive or corporate boutique visits to clients (Kumar & Shah, 2004).

Health service firms must continually ask themselves, who is our target market? This is because there are individual differences, and every customer has a need which could be totally different or almost the same as others. Customers are sophisticated, and they may want different values from the firm. Therefore, companies should know their segment of the target market and place great emphasis on the requests and desires of their customers, so as to fit within the firms' value proposition. According to Brodie, Hollebeek, Jurić, and Ilić (2011), new customers are difficult to secure at a mature stage in their life cycles. It is very difficult when customers retained by firms switch to competitors. Employees in the firm play a paramount role in targeting the right customers, so firms must consider how growing the number of service employees will enable them to meet the expectations of some specific categories of customers, as in their personal style and practical capability. Some firms do not consider the value their targeted customers will get from them but instead, concentrate more on the number of customers they need to acquire. When this happens, the firm will not be able to know the right customers they need to serve, which can lead to customer dissatisfaction and disloyalty.

Targeting the right customers is essential to service delivery because the right customers will most likely remain devoted to the health enterprises for longer, and also will spread word-of-mouth advertising to others. They are also more likely to act as marketers of the firm, which then leads to value addition to the firm. Targeting and obtaining the precise customers will bring in long-lasting proceeds, constant development from recommendations, and customer retention.

The starting point of raising loyal or faithful customers begins with the firm's ability to target the right customers. Targeting the right customers starts with the appropriate segmentation of the market. This aids a firm to choose a target audience which its services can be designed to satisfy effectively. However, deciding on which segment of the market to focus on is a challenging task for most firms in the service industry, since they have to adopt both a market focus and a service focus (Khoo-Lattimore & Prayag, 2015).

Health businesses could be selective when they segment what they are actually looking for in the right customer, if they want to build and maintain effective relationships with their customers. This means that firms should concentrate on obtaining customers who will be aligned and suitable for their principal value scheme. Corresponding customers to the companies' proficiencies is vigorous. Leaders need to reason cautiously to determine in what manner consumer desires correspond to the health service firm's operational components, such as swiftness and service excellence. Firms also ought to take into consideration how well their service facility workforces will be able to encounter and interact with their exact categories of customers, in terms of individual elegance and practical proficiency.

## Analyzing and Managing Customer Databases

Analyzing and managing a customer database is one thing that every health service enterprise should look at, in order to promote a relationship that will go a long way for both the customers and the firm. The reason is that analysis of customers' commitment provides enterprises with the opportunity to provide good treatment to their individual customers, implying that the treatment given one client will be different from that given to another, according to Ryals (2008). Nevertheless, customers are progressively placing additional importance on the eminence of the goods consumed other than what they pay for, and this is not far from the truth of goods that are not consumable, (Garcia-Murillo & Annabi, 2002). Therefore, firms should know what their clients want, so that the necessary resources can be allocated to satisfy the needs of their clients (Fang, Tsai, & Chang, 2005).

According to Probst, Romhardt, and Raub (2000), firms that would want to enhance the quality of their service should put their clients at the forefront as a salient resource of information. Hereafter, companies ought to constantly inspire sound discourses among other subdivisions of the firm and employees in other and diverse settings, in order for all and sundry to part information and interrelate with other members, to generate new ideas (Castaneda & Rios, 2008; Värlander, 2008). Therefore, service marketers need to create consciousness about what people want, about excellence, worth, presentation, and other performance metrics; and persuade buyers who are most interested and cheer their buying choices. For successful management of customer base, there should be good communication. Superior communication grounded on sound positioning is a more promising lever for competitive advantage (Fischer, 2014). This is because it aids to retain displeased consumers well-versed in activities to resolve glitches (Ndubisi & Kok Wah, 2005). Once there is an active rapport between the organization and its customers, consumers are healthier and conversant with the firm's creativities and doings, thus decreasing ambiguity and increasing the quality of their association. Hence, marketers need to adopt a tactical attitude to customer retention. Retaining customers is possible when the organization develops a very long-lasting, less costly relationship with customers for the common advantage of both.

While the quality of health service needs to be improved by looking for new ways to realign service to customers' needs, corporations need to work strategically to obtain the client data required to give suggestions for service improvements that can be used to fulfill customers' needs and wants (Qin & Prybutok, 2009). Therefore, firms ought to inaugurate active conduits by which to obtain clients information that will help them expand the client's connections, so as to develop the quality of service. Hence, firms must segment their market so as to know the level of their customers in relations to their purchase behavior as well as their obligation levels. This will allow the firm to tailor goods and manage the customers according to their commitment levels. It will also give the firm the idea of how and where their profit is coming from, whether from their top-level customers or lower-level customers. Different customer levels should be treated with different service expectations and needs. This is why it is very prudent for the firm to analyze and manage its customer base to be able to appreciate the requirements of its customers and regulate their way of servicing customers subsequently.

A crucial aspect of any health firm's positioning strategy will be to form relationships to strengthen its position, in one or more networks. Astute management of a health service institution's customer and competitor databases (and by extension, relationships), could help greatly in this regard. Burt (1992) has argued that it is these relationships and accompanying social structures that render competition imperfect by creating entrepreneurial opportunities for some players and not for others. Social capital (as distinct from financial and human capital) in terms of the players' relationships with other players, both within and beyond the firm, makes it possible for a player to get a higher rate of return on investment (Burt, 1992).

## Building Customer Loyalty

Healthcare institutions cannot function without customers (Bruhn & Homburg, 2008), and it is increasingly insufficient to barely meet the needs of these customers. The firm needs to develop a lifelong association with them to make the healthcare firm profitable. There is, therefore, a shift to a relationship perspective of transacting a business, where the firm places emphasis on retaining current clients and improving each clients' purchases (Bruhn & Homburg, 2008; Pop & Pelau, 2006). Healthcare firms need to make sure they meet customers' demands as this will enable them to develop firm devotees, which may last a lifetime. The idea is that clients whose needs are not met could abandon their healthcare provider for a competitor.

Clients get committed when they become loyal. Commitment refers to modification procedures, which are the end products of each side's drift to act and demonstrate good behavior towards the other. This brings about a healthcare firm's connection with its clients. An example is the presence of links between the client and the firm. These links serve as switching barriers since building customer loyalty is not an easy task. Since the hospital market is competitive, building customer loyalty can be a challenge to hospitals unless they place emphasis on patient satisfaction (Jones & Sasser, 1995). Providers must not only maintain high clinical standards, but also services that satisfy the patients. The healthcare firm has to do this by targeting and attracting the right customers, and making sure that they deliver to the satisfaction of their targeted customers. The main objective of every healthcare firm is usually to stay profitable, and one way of achieving this is to attract, keep, and retain committed clients. Building client commitment is essential to healthcare service delivery. Building customer loyalty comes with many benefits such as creating and retaining committed customers who then refer others to the firm.

According to Kumar and Shah (2004), there are two types of customer loyalty which are behavioral and attitudinal loyalty. With attitudinal loyalty, customers show likelihood or attitudes of futuristic purchase and recommendations to friends, family, colleagues; while in behavioral loyalty, the customer does an actual purchase and increases the firm's monetary value. In other words, while behavioural loyalty results in purchase, attitudinal loyalty might end up in acknowledgement, recommendations or a few likes and comments on social media which may someday amount to an actual purchase. Nonetheless, it is imperative for a brand to build both categories of loyal customers as one produces positive word-of-mouth, and another increases monetary value. A healthcare company is able to minimize cost greatly by developing a positive connection with clients and retaining them. For instance, it has been proven that it is less costly to deal with current clients than to gain and deal with new ones (Ndubisi, 2006). When there is a good relationship with customers, firms can also reduce the uncertainty of demand by building connections with clients. Trust is an important relationship and marketing ingredient. It convinces the client's foreseeable and mandatory attitude/behavior as far as the other party is concerned. Thus, a comparatively elevated assurance is joined to later returns. Accomplishing promises sometimes improves customers' confidence in the institution, thereby, increasing the value of bonds between them (Ndubisi & Kok Wah, 2005). An enterprise ought to develop accurate plans aimed at targeting the exact customer base they want, and find ways to strategically execute this plan in their marketing. Building customer loyalty involves a series of processes, that is, the firm must capture the hearts and minds of customers, target prospects with precision, take care of what they want, give customers the chance to do the talking, challenge them to become better, and seek the progress and welfare of their customers.

Since every healthcare firm wants to build customer loyalty, its products and services should look attractive and reflect the thoughts of its customers.

The goods and services should engage customer's imaginations. The firm should design products and services to attract value propositions and produce genuine customer interest. They should ensure that there is flawless execution on the promises they make, by providing customers with solid evidence of their reliability. Again, healthcare firms must appreciate who their right customers are, and pay attention to them with exactness. Firms should not just focus on attracting a large volume of customers, but should also get the right ones and focus on them, this is essential to the growth and building of customer loyalty. Examining the customers' needs and satisfying those needs, helps in retaining them. Healthcare firms can effectively monitor their customers to determine how they use their products and track any problems associated with the health products that could cause customers to back out. Healthcare firms should be proactive to correct any problem and save the relationship that they have with customers.

Another way to build customer loyalty is to manage the experience, not just the products or services they have at hand. Firms should track in what means and how well they can convey their assurances to their clients on points because it is very vital to the frontrunners' method of handling the client's bond and building loyalty. Anything customers go through daily when they come into connections with the firm defines the value of the constant association. Normally, customers expect the completion of their task to be error-free, that is, with no problem. So, the healthcare firm should have active interactions with customers to reshape what customers perceive about the services delivered and help to strengthen client faithfulness. Customers should also be allowed to do the talking. Healthcare firms should have an active interaction with customers, get to know their opinion, and use what they find to correct any shortcomings. This will help to deliver fine-tuned product offerings to their targeted audiences. Healthcare customers should be given a chance to provide feedback on the quality of experience they encounter with the healthcare firm.

Patients-loyalty is a critical success factor for any healthcare provider, as loyal patients are likely to return to the same healthcare provider, spread positive word-of-mouth, and recommend the provider to others. However, building patient loyalty is a difficult process in healthcare. First, healthcare providers should focus on service quality and deliver high-quality services that generate satisfied customers. Satisfaction is one of the main drivers of patient loyalty. Patients who are satisfied with the quality of their interactions with hospital staff are more likely to take treatments for similar and different medical problems and recommend the provider to their relatives and friends (Chahal, 2008). Empathy (i.e., the ability to understand the thoughts, feelings, or emotions of patients) and assurance (i.e., the extent to which healthcare providers are knowledgeable, courteous, and able to inspire trust and confidence), positively influence patients' willingness to return to hospitals (Anbori, Ghani, Yadav, Daher, & Su, 2010; Ramli & Sjahruddin, 2015). Kitapci, Akdogan, and Dortyol (2014) indicate that empathy and assurance positively influence patient loyalty through satisfaction. Hospitals can focus on brand image that enhances patient loyalty (Wu, 2011).

## Customer Relationship Management in Healthcare Delivery

Healthcare marketers should not only design quality products but also products that are tailored to meet the requirements of the consumers. To be able to accomplish this, a healthcare organization needs to design a customer-centric plan to help ascertain healthcare consumers' needs and the services that will fill the individual's desires. Customer targeting is an important ingredient of customer relationship marketing (CRM), as it is a way to determine the few reliable customers situated in the lots of potential customers, as well as to retain these customers (Woo et al., 2005). Initially, the emergence of CRM was a result of the switch from traditional marketing to relationship marketing. Earlier in the 2000s, focusing on customers was still a newly emerging thought and was regarded as the foundation of CRM (Bolton, 2004; Bose, 2002). At the core of customer-centric orientation was the desire in using CRM software to design a long-lasting connection with consumers to service them better, according to Stefanou, Sarmaniotis, and Stafyla (2003) and Rigby and Ledingham (2004).

Managing customer affiliation is usually seen when the administration of jointly advantageous interactions is taken into consideration (LaPlaca, 2004), and where the customer's information is given the most attention (Verhoef & Langerak, 2002). At this stage, there usually appears to be a general implication which indicates that acquiring technical know-how would aid the organization in customer interactions (Campbell, 2003; Dewhurst, Martinez Lorente, & Dale, 1999; Karimi, Somers, & Gupta, 2001). But slowly the investigation or study into CRM emerged under many umbrellas leading to a divided set of ways, meanings, and findings. The focus on organizations was replaced by an emphasis on consumer-research, centered on firms' activities of managing customer relationship, such as segmenting the market, targeting, and cross-selling (Ryals, 2005). Organizations used customer information for their own reasons, considering it to be the property of the enterprise, and losing the focus on clients. The tactical way or approach to CRM conceptualizes it as a procedure, a way of thinking, of competence, or technical know-how (Zablah, Bellinger, & Johnston, 2004). The tactical way of CRM is all about relating personally to the individual customer, and also eventually, optimizing a very long-lasting and significant relationship between the individual customer and the firm, as Peppard (2000) stressed.

According to Peppers and Rogers (2011) in the recent professional atmosphere, "Every company ought to be implementing good customer approaches earlier or far ahead with changing degrees of eagerness and accomplishment" (p. 7). Usually, two reasons arise from this: Customers desire a personal engagement, and as an elaborate systematic plan of action, it is a productive way of transacting business. In reality, strategic CRM has so many ways of "improving shareholder value through the development of appropriate relationships with key customers and customer segments" (Payne & Frow, 2004, 2005, p. 268). This involves the cohort of customer information, finding out who the most profitable customers are, improving customer loyalty by engaging with the customers, and offering tailored goods and services produced at the same period by minimizing cost (Cao & Gruca, 2005; Rigby, Reichheld, & Schefter, 2002). Commencing from the tactical standpoint, the main clue to managing customer interconnections is to generate systematic plans of action to fascinate (the exact) clients, and also optimize their long-lasting worth through nurturing the loyalty levels of the clients. It is about getting, fostering, supervising, as well as keeping clients, and that is the reason CRM emphasizes the value of connecting schemes and procedures that can be used to recognize customers, produce customer awareness, strengthen customer affiliations, and create customer ideas of the organizations' offerings. Premeditated client relationship management (CRM) ought to be regarded as the IDIC-model that is isolating, distinguishing, interrelating, and customizing (Peppers & Rogers, 2004, 2011), by underlining the appropriate value to a fruitful CRM stratagem of identifying the accurate customers at the initial stage.

Furthermore, strategic CRM should clearly define how an organization should effectively engage with its customers as it has been realized that customers' requirements will continue to vary. As a result, client's affiliation management structures have a duty to evolve and enhance, in order to give consumers desirable products and services and in turn retain clients for the firm. Customers understand that when CRM is implemented appropriately, it is able to give a coordinated network that aids in the tailoring and individualizing of their needs. If a firm successfully sustains exuberance and customer involvement, and also progressively merges transactions marketing and caring for the clients, then it is likely to augment consumer commitment and extend customer retention time (Chalmeta, 2006; King & Burgess, 2008; Ozgener & Iraz, 2006).

Customer relationship management (CRM) is defined as individualizing a company's means by personalizing its goods and services, and by doing so, the enterprise can optimally satisfy client needs and thereby generate a very long-lasting faithfulness when it comes to relationships (Garrido-Moreno & Padilla-Meléndez, 2011). CRM allows a firm to understand, segment, and target their right customers. It also helps the company to come to a realization that its customers want to defect or have any problems to which attention must be paid. It will also help the firm to identify the customer's lifetime value, which implies that the company evaluated each person by considering the customer's possible repeat or future purchases and by assessing individual customer-level marketing costs. According to Verhoef and Lemon (2013), firms can also obtain a distinct forecast for customer worth if there is appropriate CRM implementation. Client relationship aims to enhance the association concerning firms and their consumers by supervising CRM agitations, such as customer recognition, attraction, preservation, and evolvement in order to improve gains (Ngai, Xiu, & Chau, 2009).

Service software is extended to filter customer data for the benefit of the customer. Most service marketers use CRM in their firms, for example, banking, telecommunication, restaurants, and many others. Many firms which adopt the CRM provide some software which provides speedy delivery and provide firms with easy tasks. The applications of CRM include data collection which adopts customer data, such as contact details and their service preferences. Customer information is not only used inside a firm to assist its worth creation, but also for customer gains. In the same vein, customer data is used, not only as a firm's capital but also as capital for customer worth creation. This brings about several business ideas that transcend the usual exchange. In addition to products, firms can provide customers with information that can support customers' value creation. It also includes data analysis which analyzes and categorizes the system according to the criteria set by the firm. This helps the firm to identify who their customers are and deliver services to them accordingly.

The CRM applications also include marketing automation, which helps to pull out customer information and makes it possible for firms to earmark their customers' strength for special purposes such as sales leads and other opportunities. CRM is slowly giving priority for customers by discovering how to nurture the likely profitability CRM could offer customers. Thereby, shifting the bearing of CRM from licensing companies to licensing customers, from the interior to the exterior, and also from looking at it as a mode of profit formation for companies, gives the firm the opportunity to fully address customers needs instead of just being sales-focused. CRM repositions the firm to embrace the shift from a product orientation to a service orientation.

According to Diller, Haas, and Ivens (2005), a healthcare firm can possess an efficient CRM scheme if it examines the six elements within the 6I's CRM model. These six elements are the information, the investment, the individualization, the interaction, the integration, and the overall idea of the concept. As stated by Diller et al. (2005), a company has to initially examine the data about the customers and their demands, and this is the only way a firm can produce personalized goods and services. To associate with the customer, it is prudent to have clarity of customer data. Just as the firm is supposed to be well-informed about its clients, the client should be equally informed about the firm's products and services; this will enable them to work successfully (Diller et al., 2005). Firms should designate and itemize the clients according to the information on hand in order to identify the most valuable clients.

For a successful customer relationship management, a firm should be able to identify the most valuable clients and devote more to them. Similarly, it should be able to identify the less valuable clients so it can minimize cost as far as these clients are concerned (Pop & Palau, 2005). Again, as stated in the 6I's model by Diller et al. (2005), one other vital facet is individualization. To be able to meet clients' demands and also enhance the association with clients, a firm requires an examination of individualized demands and choices, particularly in the business-to-business sector. It is prudent to examine the specialities of the manufacturing process and the needs of the clients; this is in order to identify the required techniques needed to adapt and merge production to individual needs. By a constant engagement with the clients, it is likely for a firm to identify its individualized demands and specialities. In reality, the client is merged in the manufacturing procedure, by being in charge of the manufacturing procedure. The final ingredient of the 6I's model by Diller et al. (2005) is the idea. It plays the role of an integrator by possessing, designing, and combining all the other five elements. It comprises of the regulation of the customer relationship management structure in the firm, by setting the management of the CRM structure, the apparatus, the characteristics, and the people in charge of the execution and the operation of the system.

Customer relationship management for healthcare, also called patient relationship management, is a system designed specifically for use by healthcare organizations to facilitate patient engagement, satisfaction, and experience, throughout the entire patient–doctor relationship. The CRM healthcare system aims to increase the quality of healthcare and the lives of patients. The system uses multiple sources of data to provide a comprehensive overview of the habits and activities of patients (Kocev & Kocev, 2019).

## Conclusion

In conclusion, the increase of the competition among healthcare firms in the world market enforces service marketing firms to devise efficient and effective client faithfulness strategies to improve the associations with clients and build customer loyalty. In other words, if there is improved service quality, it affects customer loyalty through relationship quality. According to Roberts, Varki, and Brodie (2003) and Bei and Chiao (2006), service quality provides added value and leads to customer loyalty only through customer satisfaction. This means there is no service quality without a good relationship. If healthcare customers feel good about the treatment they get from their service providers, they are expected to perceive an advanced quality of services rendered, and they will be more willing to enter an extensive and lasting bond with the enterprise. Also, the model by Diller et al. (2005) is a good roadmap of what a firm ought to do, so that they can retain their healthcare customers for competitive advantage, as well as to upsurge their fulfillment. If the firm attains additional knowledge of its customers, it will also get the mandate to act on this knowledge in an added effectiveness and well-organized way. With the 6I model as a guide to managing relationships and building loyalty, service marketing firms would also have the chance to employ the CRM approach in different means that would increase the performance of a firm. Utilizing customer relationship management (CRM) in service delivery will also provide an exclusive opportunity for enterprises in scheming and in executing the bond of customer tactics. However, healthcare marketing firms should reflect all of the rudiments if the healthcare enterprise wants to improve its relationship with their customers for a long-lasting bond.

## Review Questions

1. Explain why targeting the right customers is essential to service delivery.
2. Discuss how to analyze and manage a healthcare institution's customer base.
3. Explain the role of a customer relationship management system in the delivery of healthcare service.

## MINI CASE-STUDY: LOSING MARKET SHARE TO A CLOSE COMPETITOR

Dr. Kwame Baba has been John Mayer's physician for years. Dr. Kwame was leaving the practice after 20 years of active service, and he recommended Dr. Shiana Williams as his replacement. John accepted the recommendation. Weeks later, John visited the clinic for an appointment with Dr. Shiana; he was the second patient to be seen that morning. A nurse showed John the waiting room, took some short notes, then left John with a smile and a stack of old magazines to wait for the doctor.

John waited for 15 minutes before he decided to inquire at the front desk about the delay. He was assured that the doctor was coming, and John returned to his seat. Thirty minutes later, he went back to the front desk expecting at least an explanation for the delay if not an apology. To his amazement, the desk nurse laughed and said: "Oh, she's always late." John didn't find this funny and remarked that being late with no explanation or concern for patients was rude. "Cancel my appointment and tell the doctor why I won't be returning to this clinic," John said, and he left. He called his friend who then recommended another clinic. John called them immediately and scheduled an appointment for that day and was attended to in less than 10 minutes.

He later learned that the average time a patient waits to see a doctor in the first clinic is 28 minutes and 35 seconds.

### Discussion Questions

1. If John had been given a reasonable explanation for the delay, an emergency with another patient, for example, what were his best options: Continue to wait? Cancel and reschedule? Alternatively, find another clinic? Offer one or two good reasons for each of those choices?
2. "Oh, she's always late." What does that say about the clinic's standards? How should the nurse have been reprimanded and what kind of training should she receive to meet a higher standard of customer service.
3. If the doctor is always late to attend to patients, it is likely that the hospital will lose patients over time. What actions would you take to correct this situation to avoid losing out to a competitor?

## References

Anbori, A., Ghani, S. N., Yadav, H., Daher, A. M., & Su, T. T. (2010). Patient satisfaction and loyalty to the private hospitals in Sana'a, Yemen. *International Journal of Quality Health Care, 22*(4), 310–315.

Bei, L. T., & Chiao, Y. C. (2006). The determinants of customer loyalty: An analysis of intangible factors in three service industries. *International Journal of Commerce and Management, 16*(3/4), 162–177.

Bolton, M. (2004). Customer centric business processing. *International Journal of Productivity and Performance Management, 53*(1), 44–51.

Bose, R. (2002). Customer relationship management: Key components for IT success. *Industrial Management & Data Systems, 102*(2), 89–97.

Brodie, R. J., Hollebeek, L. D., Jurić, B., & Ilić, A. (2011). Customer engagement: Conceptual domain, fundamental propositions, and implications for research. *Journal of Service Research, 14*(3), 252–271.

Bruhn, M., & Homburg, C. (2008). *Handbook: Customer relationship management.* Wiesbaden, Germany: Gabler.

Burt, R. (1992). The social structure of competition. In N. Nohria & R. Eccles (Eds.), *Networks and organizations: Structure, form, and action* (pp. 57–91). Cambridge, MA: Harvard Business Review Press.

Campbell, A. J. (2003). Creating customer knowledge competence: Managing customer relationship management programs strategically. *Industrial Marketing Management, 32*(5), 375–383.

Cao, Y., & Gruca, T. S. (2005). Reducing adverse selection through customer relationship management. *Journal of Marketing, 69*(4), 219–229.

Castaneda, D. I., & Rios, M. F. (2008). From individual learning to organizational learning. *The Electronic Journal of Knowledge Management, 5*(4), 363–372.

Chahal, H. (2008). Predicting patient loyalty and service quality relationship: A case study of Civil Hospital, Ahmedabad, India. *Vision, 12*(4), 45–55.

Chalmeta, R. (2006). Methodology for customer relationship management. *Journal of Systems and Software, 79*(7), 1015–1024.

Copulsky, J. R., & Wolf, M. J. (1990). Relationship marketing: Positioning for the future. *Journal of Business Strategy, 11*(4), 16–20.

Dagger, T. S., Danaher, P. J., & Gibbs, B. J. (2009). How often versus how long: The interplay of contact frequency and relationship duration in customer-reported service relationship strength. *Journal of Service Research, 11*(4), 371–388.

Dewhurst, F., Martínez Lorente, A. R., & Dale, B. G. (1999). Total quality management and information technologies: An exploration of the issues. *International Journal of Quality & Reliability Management, 16*(4), 392–406.

Diller, H. Haas, A., & Ivens, B. (2005). *Sales and customer management.* Stuttgart, Germany: Kohlhammer.

Fang, S. C., Tsai, F. S., & Chang, K. C. (2005). Knowledge sharing routines, task efficiency, and team service quality in instant service-giving settings. *Journal of American Academy of Business, 6*(1), 62–67.

Fischer, S. (2014). Hospital positioning and integrated hospital marketing communications: State-of-the-art review, conceptual framework, and research agenda. *Journal of Nonprofit & Public Sector Marketing, 26*(1), 1–34.

García-Murillo, M., & Annabi, H. (2002). Customer knowledge management. *Journal of the Operational Research Society, 53*(8), 875–884.

Garrido-Moreno, A., & Padilla-Meléndez, A. (2011). Analyzing the impact of knowledge management on CRM success: The mediating effects of organizational factors. *International Journal of Information Management, 31*(5), 437–444.

Gibbert, M., Leibold, M., & Probst, G. (2002). Five styles of customer knowledge management, and how smart companies use them to create value. *European Management Journal, 20*(5), 459–469.

Godfrey, A., Seiders, K., & Voss, G. B. (2011). Enough is enough! The fine line in executing multichannel relational communication. *Journal of Marketing, 75*(4), 94–109.

Jones, T. O., & Sasser, W. E., Jr. (1995, November–December). Why satisfied customers defect. *Harvard Business Review, 73*, 88–99.

Karimi, J., Somers, T. M., & Gupta, Y. P. (2001). Impact of information technology management practices on customer service. *Journal of Management Information Systems, 17*(4), 125–158.

Keller, K. L., & Lehmann, D. R. (2006). Brands and branding: Research findings and future priorities. *Marketing science, 25*(6), 740–759.

Khoo-Lattimore, C., & Prayag, G. (2015). The girlfriend getaway market: Segmenting accommodation and service preferences. *International Journal of Hospitality Management, 45*, 99–108.

King, S. F., & Burgess, T. F. (2008). Understanding success and failure in customer relationship management. *Industrial Marketing Management, 37*(4), 421–431.

Kitapci, O., Akdogan, C., Dortyol, I. T. (2014). The impact of service quality dimensions on patient satisfaction, repurchase intentions and word-of-mouth communication in the public healthcare industry. *Procedia Social and Behavioral Sciences, 148*, 161–169.

Kocev, S., & Kocev, D. (2019). Customer relationship management in health organization. *Knowledge International Journal, 30*(6), 1691–170.

Kumar, V., & Shah, D. (2004). Building and sustaining profitable customer loyalty for the 21st century. *Journal of Retailing, 80*(4), 317–329.

LaPlaca, P. J. (2004). Letter from the editor: Special issue on customer relationship marketing. *Industrial Marketing Management, 33*(6), 463–464.

Lee, R. P., Naylor, G., & Chen, Q. (2011). Linking customer resources to firm success: The role of marketing program implementation. *Journal of Business Research, 64*(4), 394–400.

Mithas, S., Krishnan, M. S., & Fornell, C. (2005). Why do customer relationship management applications affect customer satisfaction? *Journal of Marketing, 69*(4), 201–209.

Naidu, G. M., Parvatiyar, A., Sheth, J. N., & Westgate, L. (1999). Does relationship marketing pay? An empirical investigation of relationship marketing practices in hospitals. *Journal of Business Research, 46*(3), 207–218.

Ndubisi, O. N. (2006). Effect of gender on customer loyalty: A relationship marketing approach. *Marketing Intelligence & Planning, 24*(1), 48–61.

Ndubisi, O. N., & Kok Wah, C. (2005). Factorial and discriminant analyses of the underpinnings of relationship marketing and customer satisfaction. *International journal of bank marketing, 23*(7), 542–557.

Ngai, E. W., Xiu, L., & Chau, D. C. (2009). Application of data mining techniques in customer relationship management: A literature review and classification. *Expert Systems With Applications, 36*(2), 2592–2602.

Özgener, Ş., & İraz, R. (2006). Customer relationship management in small–medium enterprises: The case of Turkish tourism industry. *Tourism Management, 27*(6), 1356–1363.

Palmatier, R. W. (2008). *Relationship marketing*. Cambridge, MA: Marketing Science Institute.

Payne, A., & Frow, P. (2004). The role of multichannel integration in customer relationship management. *Industrial Marketing Management, 33*(6), 527–538.

Payne, A., & Frow, P. (2005). A strategic framework for customer relationship management. *Journal of Marketing, 69*(4), 167–176.

Peppard, J. (2000). Customer relationship management (CRM) in financial services. *European Management Journal, 18*(3), 312–327.

Peppers, D., & Rogers, M. (2004). *Managing customer relationships. A strategic framework*. Hoboken, NJ: Wiley.

Peppers, D., & Rogers, M. (2011). *Managing customer relationships. A strategic framework* (2nd ed.). Hoboken, NJ: Wiley.

Pop, N. A., & Pelau, C. (2005). Controlling elements in marketing. Evaluation methods of customers. In *Revista de Management şi Inginerie Economică, 4*(3), 43–52.

Probst, G., Romhardt, K., & Raub, S. (2000). *Managing knowledge: Building blocks for success*. New York, NY: Wiley.

Qin, H., & Prybutok, V. R. (2009). Service quality, customer satisfaction, and behavioral intentions in fast-food restaurants. *International Journal of Quality and Service Sciences, 1*(1), 78–95.

Ramli A. H., & Sjahruddin, H. (2015). Building patient loyalty in healthcare services. *International Review of Management and Business Research, 4*(2), 391–401.

Reibstein, D. J., Day, G., & Wind, J. (2009). Guest editorial: Is marketing academia losing its way? *Journal of Marketing, 73*(4), 1–3.

Rigby, D. K., & Ledingham, D. (2004). *CRM done right. Harvard Business Review, 82*(11), 118–129.

Rigby, D. K., Reichheld, F. F., & Schefter, P. (2002). Avoid the four perils of CRM. *Harvard Business Review, 80*(2), 101–109.

Roberts, K., Varki, S., & Brodie, R. (2003). Measuring the quality of relationships in consumer services: An empirical study. *European Journal of marketing, 37*(1/2), 169–196.

Ryals, L. (2005). Making customer relationship management work: The measurement and profitable management of customer relationships. *Journal of Marketing, 69*(4), 252–261.

Ryals, L. (2008). Determining the indirect value of a customer. *Journal of Marketing Management, 24*(7–8), 847–864.

Sheth, J. N., & Parvatiyar, A. (1995, Fall). Relationship marketing in consumer markets: Antecedents and consequences. *Journal of the Academy of Marketing Science, 23*(4), 255–271.

Stefanou, C. J., Sarmaniotis, C., & Stafyla, A. (2003). CRM and customer-centric knowledge management: An empirical research. *Business Process Management Journal, 9*(5), 617–634.

Värlander, S. (2008). The role of situated embodied interaction in the banking customer knowledge creation process. *International Journal of Knowledge Management, 4*(4), 62–76.

Verhoef, P. C., & Langerak, F. (2002). Eleven misconceptions about customer relationship management. *Business Strategy Review, 13*(4), 70–76.

Verhoef, P. C., & Lemon, K. N. (2013). Successful customer value management: Key lessons and emerging trends. *European Management Journal, 31*(1), 1–15.

Woo, J. Y., Bae, S. M., & Park, S. C. (2005). Visualization method for customer targeting using customer map. *Expert Systems with Applications, 28*(4), 763–772.

Wu, C. C. (2011). The impact of hospital brand image on service quality, patient satisfaction and loyalty. *African Journal of Business Management, 5*(12), 4873–4882.

# 12

## *Marketing Tool Kit for Healthcare Managers*

### Chapter Outline

- Introduction
- The Tool Kit
- The Motivation
- The Market
- Customer Relationship Management
- Medical Stakeholders
- Non-Medical Stakeholders
- Brand Development
- Advertising and Marketing Communication
- Content Creation
- Conclusion

*Marketing in Healthcare-Related Industries,* pages 265–273

## Chapter Outcome

By the end of this chapter, the reader will be able to

- explain the various tool kits and why they are relevant for startups,
- explain why it is important to identify the key players in the business sector,
- discuss how social media contents can influence target customers, and
- discuss the relevance of branding to a firm.

## Introduction

Strategic planning describes the direction a firm should go to respond to the opportunities and challenges of the marketplace. No doubt, there are opportunities within this industry, and a firm needs to be rightly positioned to seize this opportunity. It is acknowledged that starting and managing a healthcare practice is not a small feat, the medical training and experience of healthcare providers cannot be overestimated; however, it is essential to understand the marketing implications on the practice and its effect towards remaining commercially viable. Even charity firms and not-for-profit healthcare firms need to make an effort to be sustainable in order to keep providing for the customers; this suggests, in addition to the healthcare and medical aspects, effective marketing management can contribute to the viability of a firm.

With the theoretical insight into healthcare management provided in the preceding chapters, this chapter aims to summarize them all with a focus on managerial implications. The chapter raises thought-provoking questions to challenge managers on actions they have taken and those they are still considering. It is important to state that this chapter may not answer any questions, but will provide insight into critical marketing strategies to consider for a healthcare firm. For marketing to be successful, organizations must be market responsive, should have a clear vision, and take actionable steps to achieve set goals. It is anticipated that this chapter will contribute towards achieving those objectives/targets.

For the sake of clarity, some assumptions will be made. Firstly, the business context which assumes that a new medical center is to be established. This center will be providing primary health and general practices. Another assumption is that they will need to formulate marketing strategies as they start operations. The medical center will be referred to as the *firm*. This illustration can also be applied to a dental practice or a veterinary practice. It is essential to understand the business context that will shape the strategic direction.

The second assumption is the practitioner's context. It is assumed that the firm was established by a medical doctor. The medical doctor will be referred to as the manager. This does not mean that a physiotherapist or a dentist cannot start the firm; it only suggests that they will be referred to as the managers in the context of this chapter. This context highlights the role of the person responsible for the strategic direction of the firm. This does not, however, imply that the manager will be responsible for everything, but a holistic understanding is essential, and after that, there can be delegations of duty for instance, someone to be responsible for the website and social media touchpoints and another for the reception desk.

The third assumption is the country context. It is assumed that the firm will be established in Africa. Healthcare provision is essential in all countries, and it is important to understand the country context and how it shapes the marketing and management strategies, especially with regards to government involvement and healthcare insurance. As discussed in Chapter 1, a typical African country operates privately funded healthcare, as there is little investment and contribution from the government. Customers often pay for their healthcare as the National Health Insurance Scheme is in a developing stage. This country context will, therefore, affect the paying capabilities of the customers.

Lastly, is the assumption termed Customer context. Businesses now operate in a value-based, consumer-driven world; it will not be surprising if patients consider themselves customers of the firm. They believe they are not only coming for treatment, but they are also bringing money, and therefore, should be treated well. Hence, in this context, the patients will be referred to as customers. Health induces a sense of affinity and the need for customer involvement. This customer context also includes family members who are supporting their relatives in making payments to the firm.

## The Tool Kit

It is essential to acknowledge that the healthcare industry is quite big and diverse. Therefore, one rule may not be applicable to all, hence, this section presents the tool kit containing different action points and questions where managers can select the right tool to deal with the strategic decision to be made. Figure 12.1 illustrates the key sections and interrelationship within the tool kit, which begins with the motivation for setting up the business (the firm).

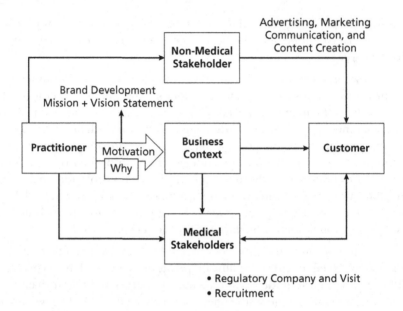

**Figure 12.1**    Marketing toolkit for healthcare managers.

## *The Motivation*

### Why Did I Start This Clinic?

It is important for the manager to highlight the motivation for starting the practice as this will shape the strategic direction. Managers should be able to answer the "why" questions, as this will feed into any marketing and advertising campaign. Why did I decide to start a new hospital in Africa? Why did I decide to start a new veterinary or dental clinic? The manager must identify what makes the firm unique to differentiate it from other players in the industry. This understanding makes the business context more tangible. Hence, the practitioner knows what business he/she is going into and must be better prepared to engage with the customers and other stakeholders. This motivation should include the need to serve the customers and provide a quality service. The mission and vision statements should be written down and well documented. This will be needed for the brand development and for engagement with non-medical stakeholders like advertising and branding agencies who will communicate with the consumers. The diversity of the industry is recognized, and therefore, the manager needs to understand where they stand in the broad spectrum of activities in order to develop and implement their marketing strategy. How is a general practice clinic different from a dental clinic? How is a residential care home for the elderly different from a rehabilitation center? This should be considered in terms of operations, regulations, and even customer base. Managers need to know what their firm stands for (mission, vision statements, and core values) and what makes it different from other healthcare providers (brand differentiation).

## *The Market*

### What Do I Know About Customers and Competitors?

With the understating of the motivation for starting the firm, the managers need to further understand the market in which they want to operate. The understanding of the market can be summed up as market research. Managers need to know their prospective customers and competitors. The firm needs to pay close attention to the operating market profile, which encompasses the market size, competitors, and stages of growth. A situational analysis of the threats and opportunities to which the firm can respond to, taking into consideration its mission, should be carried out.

Additionally, managers must endeavor to understand their target customer preferences. Firms should generally strive to gain an understanding of what their customers want in order to build connections. This involves setting up a customer relationship management system (next stage in the tool kit). By doing this, healthcare companies can collect information on how customers spend money, find out what customers want, and subsequently make predictions on what customers may demand. The understanding of the market will shape the advertising and marketing communication, ensuring the customers can engage with the message.

## *Customer Relationship Management*

### How Best Can I Relate to My Customers?

With the understanding of the market, managers need to engage with the customer. Acknowledging the country context, the African customers will have a different expectation from the Western customers who have the option of both government and private funded healthcare provision. Managers should be mindful of different touch points as they relate with customers. The frontline staff needs to be carried along as well. These touch points, including the website, telephone enquiries, and first visit to the firm offers the opportunity to collect valuable information about the customers and relate with them better. The touch point experience describes total customer experience.

Managers should consider investing in a customer management system which helps save time and meets the business needs. The firm should be able to manage interaction with current and prospective customers as the system should be able to organize appointments and reminders, email marketing, task management, and marketing automation integration. Customers should be reminded about an appointment, perhaps through text messages and emails while newsletters and relevant information could be sent through automated emails. Customers should have the opportunity to engage with the firm as well; this suggests the need for active communication channels, importantly through the website and social media. Customer relationship management should specifically focus on customer retention that will ultimately be driving sales growth. Even though customers' information may be used for marketing purposes, health records should be securely kept and automatically backed up.

## Medical Stakeholders

### Who Am I Dealing Within This Sector?

The market has different players, among which are the stakeholders. This tool kit builds on Chapter 7, where the key stakeholders in healthcare provision were identified. It was noted that stakeholders in a healthcare marketing process are crucial because success and the continued existence of the firm depend on their participation and involvement. Managers need to understand the key players within the sector, and this can vary across different countries. This also involves working with the regulators, making sure the firm abides by all the regulations as an offense in that regard may affect the brand reputation and customers' trust in the firm.

## Non-Medical Stakeholders

### Who Can I Contact to Deal With Non-Medical Tasks?

Managers must recognize the need for non-medical stakeholders as they make an effort towards marketing their healthcare business. It will not be surprising that the manager may not have vast marketing experiences, with the implication that the company may not be able to implement the marketing strategy. It is, therefore, essential to work with other professionals to effectively manage the firm. Thus, this tool kit includes working with architects and interior decorators to make sure the layout and interior are functional and appealing and has the right ambience for the target audience. In understanding the business context, the design and layout of a hospital clinic should be different from a residential home for the elderly. As one of the touch points, the firm should be welcoming, appear modern, and warm. The first impression is essential as it can shape the overall evaluation of the service. Advertising and branding agencies should ensure the brand identities and marketing messages are well-communicated. Digital marketing professionals should work on using competitive keywords on web pages. They should also use inbound and outbound links in blogs. It is desirable to have a consultant to outline and ensure compliance with the regulations that are specific to the business context. This tool kit is all about getting the right people with the right set of skills to work on different parts of the strategic plan.

## Brand Development

### What Should Our Logo Represent?

Managers need to work towards building their brand as they enter the sector. This tool kit starts with brand positioning. Building on the motivation behind the firm as provided by the manager, the brand values, mission, and vision should be made available and well-integrated. The firm must be particular about differentiating itself by creating, communicating, and maintaining unique features that its valuable customers will notice. Likewise, brand identities are essential. This tool kit also raises a question about the firm's name. Will it just be called XYZ Health Practice or Red Dove Health Center, or Africa's Health Center? What will be the logo of this firm? Will it be the snake and cross, the map of Africa, or a stethoscope? What will be the brand color? Blue or red? How about the typography? What font are we using for our logo and stationeries? Considering healthcare provision to be an intangible service, an icon or character could be developed to personalize the services. This could be a red dove soft toy (related to the brand name) that could be given to children who come visiting. It can also be further developed into merchandise and souvenirs. These concepts and integrations are fundamental and suggest the need to work with professionals. As part of building the brand reputation, star ratings and other rating systems online such as Trustpilot can be used to help customers make informed decisions. Hospitals can enhance their brand image by focusing on effective customer relationship management in order to improve brand loyalty and brand awareness.

## Advertising and Marketing Communication

### How Will Customers Know What We Offer?

The firm needs patronage to remain viable, and therefore, it is essential that they make their services known to prospective customers. This awareness can be achieved through advertising. It is, therefore, essential to consider the advertising strategies to use. Will these be emotionally or rationally appealing? Do we frame the message positively or negatively? Do we use historical or statistical information? Do we need a billboard, or do we distribute handbills within the neighborhood? Do we need a TV or radio? Where can we target our customers and with what message? It is important to note that for healthcare providers, some advertising appeal may not be suitable. Likewise, advertising regulations in the country need to be considered as well; perhaps some countries will not allow healthcare firms to advertise their services. For example, direct-to-consumer advertising of prescription drugs, the different types of promotional efforts employed by pharmaceutical companies to provide prescription drug information to the general public through consumer-oriented media, is allowed currently only in the United States and New Zealand. In addition to the advertising strategies, with the understanding of the target customers, word-of-mouth and referral are essential. They can refer their friends and families. Another form of marketing is reaching out to existing customers with the different service offerings, telling them what the firm offers as they may not know that is what they need until they see the firm offers it. Testimonials can be used on the advertising campaign where the firm shares comments of those who have experienced quality service. This could be shared on social media, in print advert, and on the website. Any personal details, however, should not be included.

---

### *Content Creation*
**What Will Our Customers Find Relevant on Social Media?**

This builds upon the advertising and marketing communications. With the growing demand for digital marketing, content creation for social media is essential. The firms must make an effort to produce content that the customers can relate with. It is essential to be strategic and consistent about this. The manager and designated person/team must understand the concept behind content creation. This tool kit suggests there should be a working plan on what and where and when to create the content. These contents could be shared on social media, blogs, and websites. The username on these platforms should be unique and consistent. Firms can check their domain and social username availability across multiple networks on websites such as namecheckr.com and checkusernames.com

With regards to content creation, the chief medical officer can create a video about a medical condition to raise awareness or to answer some frequently asked questions. The team members can also be featured, and in some cases, provided the customer remain anonymous, a medical procedure can be shared. These will provide the customers and prospective customers insights into the firm and showcase their level of competence, and in turn, build more customer engagement. Also, a newsletter providing medical assistance or relevant media information and advice can be shared through emails, and if printed, made available at the reception or even shared on social media.

The role of a website as a hub for the created content cannot be over-estimated. Websites, especially mobile-enabled sites, are critical. Customers should be able to see what the firm offers; see the contact details; read more about the firm, testimonials, and the management; and book and cancel appointments. Efforts should be made at growing the email list, asking visitors to subscribe to relevant health information and contents. It should also connect to mobile map applications so that customers can find their way to the hospital. Firms should endeavor to claim their listings and location on Google map as well as provide their business information.

## Conclusion

This chapter provides practical and managerial insights into healthcare marketing management in emerging markets. Importantly, the chapter highlights some key consideration for the firm as they enter the African business terrain. The country context is essential as the firm needs to understand and engage effectively with their customers. Additionally, the firm must be aware of the stakeholders and their competitors. In an era of hyper-competition, competitive differentiation is at the heart of marketing strategy. A competitive analysis is needed to help assist the manager in understanding how to gather and analyze information about its customers, competitors, and the market.

The firm needs to identify their target audience and target them appropriately across various media. Targeting the right customers is essential to service delivery, because the right customers will most likely remain committed to the health enterprise and will spread positive word-of-mouth recommendations to others. Significantly as well, these marketing strategies need to be evaluated. As a lot of money would have been spent, the returns on investment, therefore, should be assessed to ascertain how well the plan is working and to identify what adjustments should be made. It is important to note that these tool kits are inexhaustible, many more detailed action plans were not included. However, an effort has been made to include the essential kits to consider with regards to marketing health services in emerging markets.

# *About the Authors*

**Robert Ebo Hinson** is a professor and head of the Department of Marketing and Entrepreneurship at the University of Ghana Business School. He is also a research associate at the University of the Free State Business School and has over a hundred scientific publications to his credit. He has also served as rector of the Perez University College in Ghana and holds two doctorate degrees. He holds a doctorate degree in International Business 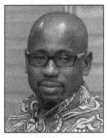 from the Aalborg University in Denmark and another in Marketing from the University of Ghana. He has consulted for and trained several institutions globally in the general areas of marketing sales and service excellence, and served as well on the boards of local and international institutions. He is also a research associate at the University of the Free State Business School, South Africa. Hinson is one of the leading voices in marketing in Africa.

**Ogechi Adeola** is an associate professor of marketing at the Lagos Business School (LBS), Pan-Atlantic University, Nigeria. She is also the academic director of LBS Sales and Marketing Academy. Her research interests include healthcare marketing, tourism and hospitality marketing, customer service management, and sales management in sub-Saharan Africa. She has published academic papers in top academic journals. Her co- 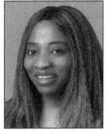 authored papers won Best Paper Awards at international conferences in

*Marketing in Healthcare-Related Industries,* pages 275–276
Copyright © 2020 by Information Age Publishing
**275**

2016–2019, consecutively. She holds a Doctorate of Business Administration (DBA) from Manchester Business School, United Kingdom and started her career at Citibank Nigeria, spending approximately 14 years in the financial sector before moving into academia. She is a coauthor of *Sales Management: A Primer for Frontier Markets,* published in 2018 by Information Age Publishing.

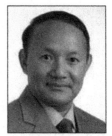

**Yam Limbu** is a professor of marketing at Montclair State University. His research interests include pharmaceutical and healthcare marketing, health communication, consumer behavior, advertising, sales, food, and nutrition. His publications have appeared in various journals, including the *British Food Journal, Health Communication, Health Education, American Journal of Health Education, International Journal of Pharmaceutical and Healthcare Marketing, Industrial Marketing Management, European Journal of Marketing, Journal of Consumer Affairs, International Journal of Advertising, Journal of Business and Industrial Marketing, International Journal of Bank Marketing,* and *Journal of Business-to-Business Marketing.* Dr. Limbu teaches pharmaceutical and healthcare marketing, marketing research, consumer behavior, and marketing analytics. He serves as the vice president of the Academy of Global Business Research and Practice. He is the editor-in-chief of the *International Journal of Business and Emerging Markets* and the *International Journal of Business and Applied Sciences.*

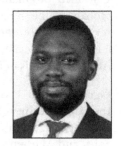

**Emmanuel Mogaji** has a PhD in marketing, and he joined the University of Greenwich in 2017 as a lecturer in advertising and marketing communications with a strong focus on service brands. He was previously at the University of Bedfordshire from 2014 to 2017 where he was an associate lecturer and a researcher at the Business and Management Research Institute. Emmanuel's primary areas of interest are ABCDE (advertising, branding, communications, digital, ethics) of marketing communications. He published peer-reviewed journal articles and book chapters and presented his works in a large number of national and international conferences. He is a fellow of the Higher Education Academy (HEA), which demonstrates his teaching philosophy and commitment to encouraging experiential learning. Emmanuel has previously worked as a marketing communication executive, responsible for creative designs and managing marketing campaigns, liaising, and building relationships with a range of stakeholders.

Printed in the United States
By Bookmasters